# How to Find a
# Four-Leaf Clover

# How to Find a Four-Leaf Clover

What Autism Can Teach Us
About Difference, Connection,
and Belonging

## Jodi Rodgers

Little, Brown Spark
New York  Boston  London

Little, Brown Spark
Hachette Book Group
1290 Avenue of the Americas, New York, NY 10104
littlebrownspark.com

First Edition: February 2024

Little, Brown Spark is an imprint of Little, Brown and Company, a division of Hachette Book Group, Inc. The Little, Brown Spark name and logo are trademarks of Hachette Book Group, Inc.

The publisher is not responsible for websites (or their content) that are not owned by the publisher.

The Hachette Speakers Bureau provides a wide range of authors for speaking events. To find out more, go to hachettespeakersbureau.com or email hachettespeakers@hbgusa.com.

Little, Brown and Company books may be purchased in bulk for business, educational, or promotional use. For information, please contact your local bookseller or the Hachette Book Group Special Markets Department at special.markets@hbgusa.com.

ISBN 9780316471978
LCCN 2023941824

Printing 1, 2023

LSC-C

Printed in the United States of America

*For Sage — guess what?*
*And for Maria — I promised.*

# Contents

### PART II

## Sharing Our Point of View:
### *Expressing and Understanding*

### PART III

## Empathizing:
### *Connecting and Belonging*

# Contents

# How to Find a
# Four-Leaf Clover

# Introduction

My grandfather taught me how to find four-leaf clovers. At the bottom of a winding rock staircase close to his home was a park filled with white-flowered clover in the early spring. I love the smell of clover. I love that it attracts the bees and that it's as soft and comforting to lie in as a quilt on a cold winter's night. I love it most because of the lessons it has taught me.

One day, as my grandfather and I walked through the clover park, he quietly said, "In amongst all of those thousands and thousands of three-leaf clovers, there are clovers that are unique. Those are the ones that you want to seek out."

When my grandfather whispered, I knew to listen and listen hard, because there was a secret coming.

"Just because you see only threes in a clover patch, don't think that everything must be the same. If you think there are only threes, you'll miss seeing the fours and the fives and even the sixes — if you're lucky. That's where the magic is."

I got on my hands and knees and studied the clover. All I could see were threes, thousands of individual threes.

"Don't look so hard, love," my grandfather said. "If you train your eyes to see the beauty in difference, it's everywhere. It's right under your nose. If you look at the world with a closed mind, all you'll see are limitations."

It's strange how some childhood lessons stick with us. A line or two of sage advice can become a recurring theme and help shape our lives in uncanny ways. For me, looking for four-leaf clovers helps me keep an open mind and reminds me that life is full of possibilities.

I never imagined that one of those possibilities would include writing a book. Up until a few years ago, that thought had never crossed my mind. This might be because the idea of spending so much time alone goes completely against my grain. My greatest happiness comes from being with other people. Finding connections with others has always brought me joy.

When I was sixteen, I was fortunate to gain work experience at a school where one of my friends' mothers taught. It was a school for children with disabilities, and I loved every second of being there, perhaps because it was the first place where I spent so much time with people who were different from me. The kids moved in a different way, communicated in a different way, and learned in a different way. My brief stint in that classroom opened my eyes to how unique we all are, and I wanted to keep learning. I wanted to know what made people tick.

My time in that school set me on a path that I have followed since. I wanted to surround myself with people who helped me view things from a new perspective. When I graduated from high school, I studied to be a teacher who works with children with disabilities, and I started working in the community and in people's homes as a disability support worker. By the time I was eighteen, I was spending many of my waking hours hanging out with people of different ages and backgrounds and who all had disabilities of one kind or another.

That was more than thirty years ago. Since then, my life has weaved through many different jobs and careers, but there's been one constant: I have always worked with autistic people.

A few years ago, I set up my own practice to provide relationship and sexuality counseling for people with disabilities. During my many years in disability support services, I had become aware that many autistic and neurodiverse people didn't have access to this type of therapy. I'm a person who thinks that relationships are the most important thing in life, so this did not sit well with me.

I had been (and still am) very happy working as a counselor, and I certainly wasn't expecting someone to call and ask me to join *Love on the Spectrum*—a TV series centered on autistic people and dating—to provide the participants with support. I definitely didn't expect the show to be so well received internationally. When I said yes to this opportunity, I didn't know that it would open so many doors, set up so many new possibilities, and create so many wonderful new friendships with the autistic people on the show.

I am not autistic. This fact created a lot of angst and trepidation for me when I began writing this book. I had to ask myself if a neurotypical person should write about autism. I struggled with this question; it consumed my thoughts. I discussed this dilemma with many of the autistic people in my life. One person, a mathematical genius, broke it down for me in an equation.

"How old were you when you first met an autistic person?" he asked. I told him. "And how old are you now?" He wrote down my answers, asked me what I had been doing each of the years between then and now, and estimated how many autistic people I had met and spent time with. The page filled with numbers and sums. "Well, by my calculations, it looks like you've met over a thousand. That's a lot of autistic people's stories you have in your head."

And when he said this, I realized that, although I wasn't a natural writer, I was a storyteller, and my life had been filled with story upon story upon story of autism: the story of the autistic person who changed my perspective on time; the person who made me rethink my relationship with objects; the person who showed me that I speak in riddles. So many tales of how autistic people changed my view of the world.

To respect people's privacy and confidentiality, I have removed the identifiers from everyone in this book. There are no real names, and none of the people in these pages are exactly like their true selves. All the individuals I'm still in contact with have read their own stories, righted my wrongs, added their perspectives, and, on a few occasions, even chosen their own pseudonyms.

One of the autistic people featured gave me the encouragement I needed to keep writing. On reading the chapter that was based on her, she sent me this text:

*I thought this was a book about autism, but it's not. It's a book about all of us.*

And she was right. Although the way that autistic people communicate and perceive the world might be different from the way neurotypical people do, these stories try to bridge the gap between "them and us." They attempt to help *all* of us have a deeper understanding of autism by offering a closer look at ourselves and the people we spend our lives with. This isn't a book about the lived experience of autism; that's not my story to tell. It's a book about what autistic people have taught me.

We all have teachers. We all have people who educate us and guide us through life. Some of these teachers are in our families or friendship groups. Some are found in schools, yoga classes, or the gym. Teachers are in churches, mosques, temples, and ashrams. They're on sports fields, in theaters, in boardrooms, and in concert halls. For myself, I have been guided to a far greater understanding of nonjudgment, compassion, empathy, humility, honesty, trust, and integrity by autistic people. I have learned about difference, connection, and belonging from my autistic teachers, and I hope that, by telling you these stories, I'll help you learn something too.

Often when I'm training or delivering workshops on disability, sexuality, and relationships, I will start by setting the audience's expectations. I will say, "You'll not find everything I say life-changing, and you will probably already know most, if not all, of what I'm going to tell you. But I hope that you can find one thing that you didn't know before and one thing that you can act upon later."

So this is the hope I have for you. I hope that within these pages, you can discover just one new thing that shifts your way of perceiving people and that, with this new knowledge, you can create better connections with those around you, whether they are neurodivergent or not.

When I started working on this book, my brother quoted Hemingway to me: "Write it as straight as you can." In keeping with this, I've tried to steer clear of jargon and academic language. But I've been very conscious of the language I use surrounding identity. Over the past three decades, I have watched the diagnostic criteria for autism be rewritten three times and revised once, and I have witnessed the language and culture of autism and disability change. When I first started working, in the 1980s, everyone used the words *autistic person* and *disabled person*. Then person-first language came into use, and for many years we used the terms *person with autism* and *person with autism spectrum disorder*, which led to the term *person on the spectrum*. In recent years this has shifted again; a large majority of the community have embraced their autistic identity and now identify as *autistic people.*

In this book I use the term *autistic person* to follow this preferred language. While I use identity-first language for autistic people, I use the term *person with a disability* for all other disabled people. This was a conscious choice, because, though I know that both identity-first and person-first language are used, there are a vast number of disabilities, and I wanted to be broad in my terminology. In saying all of this, I recognize that a person's identity is completely their own. If you call yourself an autistic person, so do I. If you call yourself a person with autism, so do I. And if you call yourself a disabled person or a person with a disability, I'll follow suit.

The book is divided into three parts. Part 1 is about how we all perceive the world and our own unique experience of thinking, sensing, and feeling. Part 2 is about how we communicate this viewpoint to others, understand one another, and express ourselves. And part 3 explores the aspects of life that connect us and give us a sense of belonging in this big, mixed-up, extraordinarily beautiful human race.

You will read about facial expressions and gestures and emotions. You'll read about trust and patience and anxiety. You'll learn about acceptance and inclusion, and you'll learn a little more about compassion. I hope this book will help you look at neurological differences from a new point of view.

My grandfather was right. When we shut our minds and see the world only from a closed perspective, when we seek only sameness and judge differences, we are not allowing ourselves the joy of all that we can learn from one another.

This book won't tell you how to find four-leaf clovers. That's between my grandfather and me. What I can tell you is that the greatest lessons and insights come from opening our minds and hearts to diversity. That was the wisdom of my grandfather.

So relax your eyes and don't look too hard. The beauty and magic found in difference is everywhere.

# Luna's Pool

L una was a pixie-like girl, fine-boned and fragile with a head that appeared too big for her seven-year-old body. She had eyes the color of mottled gray clouds on an overcast day and a shock of wispy blond hair that often stood on end, as if an electric current ran through her. Every Saturday morning, I would pick up Luna from Stanley Hall, a housing complex for people with developmental disabilities. It was a cluster of red-brick buildings surrounded by a wire fence adjacent to a major road.

On the day I met Luna, all I knew was that she didn't speak, that she loved the water, and that she had something called autism. I was only eighteen and had no knowledge of autism beyond the occasional movie reference, but I *did* know that I wanted to work with people with disabilities. As a step toward this goal, I had recently started a job as a disability support worker while studying for an undergraduate degree in education.

My job was to take Luna out on Saturday afternoons. We could do whatever we wanted from one till four, and since both of us loved water, I thought going for a swim would be the perfect plan. A local special-education school had a hydrotherapy pool that wasn't used on the weekends, and the principal had given me permission to use it. All I had to do was pick up the keys from the nuns who lived in a convent at the rear of the school.

On that first day, Luna screamed for the entire twenty-minute drive from Stanley Hall to the pool. It was a scream of deep pain and torment, and it didn't stop. Twenty minutes of screaming and thrashing and kicking and sweating, and I had nothing to offer. I didn't know how to soothe or calm her. I tried talking to her from the driver's seat while she screamed and raged in the back. I tried singing, but the screaming only got worse. I felt helpless and hopeless and in way over my head. I had no idea what Luna was doing or why she was doing it, no idea what was hurting her or causing this fear.

I ran as fast as I could to collect the keys from the convent. An elderly nun answered the door. She seemed oblivious to the anguished sounds coming from the back seat of my car. I told her that I needed the keys to the pool, and I needed them *now*.

"How lovely that you're taking a little kiddie for a dip," she said calmly, moving like molasses. She clearly was in no rush. It took everything in my power not to force my way into the convent and snatch the keys from her wrinkled hands.

When I finally had them, I raced back to the car and drove the short distance to the building that housed the pool. Luna kept screaming. I parked just outside of the pool's locked door. Luna kept screaming. I opened the car door and unbuckled her seat belt. Luna kept screaming. I lifted her out of the car seat. Luna kept screaming. I tried to lead her to the pool door, but when I touched her, she screamed even more. Getting that key in that lock was pure torture. I fumbled and swore and pleaded.

But when I finally wrenched that door open, everything changed.

Before us was a pool—twelve by thirty feet of liquid heaven. There was a single ramp that led into the water at one end with a steel handrail trailing into the depths. A pool cover was mounted at the edge of the other end like giant blue Bubble Wrap, twisted around a roller. It was just like any pool you would see in a yard, back when most pools were simple rectangles and not the curved oases that make gardens feel like the beaches of Bali or Hawaii that you see today.

It didn't matter that the room was humid and hot and there was an overpowering smell of chlorine that burned your nostrils. It didn't matter that the only fresh air entering this steamy space came from slatted windows so high up they almost touched the ceiling, as if they'd been installed as an afterthought. All that mattered was the pool. To Luna, this small rectangle of blue surrounded by rough brick walls was bliss.

I took in the pool with my eyes, but Luna examined this haven with her tongue. She ran in and licked every surface. She licked the red bricks of the walls, the metal of the handrail, the plastic of the pool cover, and the water itself, lapping at it.

At first, I was horrified. *She can't lick the pool,* I thought. *Surely this is not okay.*

But she laughed.

So I laughed.

We were not sharing this laugh; we were laughing separately, Luna in joy and me out of pure relief that the screaming had stopped.

I watched her build a relationship with this space, licking every surface. She giggled and immersed herself in the warmth of the water, then pulled herself along the edge of the pool, hand over hand, licking and making friends with each tile. She spent time with the filter and cover and skipped around the edges of the pool, making contact with all of those red bricks with her tongue.

That first day, we kept our distance from each other. I was scared of Luna's screaming, and Luna was scared of me. But the next week we went to the pool again. And the week after that. And the week after that.

Every Saturday — same time, same place, same convent run to pick up the key from the nuns. And the same licking, but with every Saturday, there was less and less screaming in the transition from one place to the other.

Every Saturday, I learned. In the oasis of the pool, I tried to get Luna to look at me, to acknowledge me, to interact with me. Initially, I did this on my terms, using a style of language and interaction that I was used to. I would call Luna's name, ask her multiple questions, and fill the air with the sound of my own voice. I tried playing games with her, floating pool toys in her direction, and throwing an inflatable ball toward her in the hope that she would pick it up and throw it back. But whenever I said her name, talked to her, or tried to get close to her, the heart-wrenching screams would begin again.

So Luna made me try a new way. A different way. Her way.

I learned that her way was all about keeping it simple and that this simplicity meant ease and calm. I learned that I didn't need to talk to her or say her name. In fact, I didn't need to speak at all. After several weeks, out of curiosity, I decided just to copy Luna. Whatever she did, I did too. I tried to clamber inside her brain and see the world as she saw it. What was she doing? What was she feeling? Why was she licking every surface?

By copying everything that Luna did, I learned that rough bricks on the tongue felt like a cat's lick on my skin. I learned that the metal of the handrail is sure and stable and provides security. I learned that each of those bubbles on the plastic pool cover was uniquely different and held its own texture and pocket of air. And I learned that water *should* be lapped, always lapped. I learned all of this with my tongue.

One Saturday, I arrived at Stanley Hall and walked to building 3 just as I'd always done. Through the glass window of that locked door, I could see Luna pacing impatiently, holding her towel and already wearing her swimsuit.

When the door buzzed, Luna came out, walked to the car, and climbed into the booster seat. She hummed to herself the whole twenty minutes of the drive.

Later, in the pool, just the two of us, lapping but not talking, Luna came up beside me and licked my arm.

We had found our connection.

### PART I

# Having a Unique Perspective

Thinking, Sensing, and Feeling

I travel a lot, both for work and for pleasure. One year I slept in thirty-two different beds over the course of forty-five nights. I hated all thirty-two. Each morning, I'd run workshops or go to meetings with bags under my eyes and my overcaffeinated heart pounding.

The first night of sleeping somewhere new is always terrible. On that first night, I'm sensitive to new noises, the creaking of the building, and the humming of the fridge. I'm aware of the lighting and the way the streetlamp casts shadows across the unfamiliar wall. I toss and turn, adjusting the pillows and occasionally punching them. I'm restless and fitful.

For the past six years, for one week a month, I've provided sexuality and relationship counseling for people with disabilities in a regional community. Every time I'm there, I stay in the same hotel. I've slept in every bed and in every room that the hotel has to offer, and they're all different. They're different shapes and sizes. The mattresses range from hard and firm to saggy and soft. Some rooms are closer to the road and some are closer to the railroad tracks, where cargo trains pass all night. Some have carpeted floors; others have polished wood or tiles. Some have big sliding doors looking out over the ocean and others have small windows with a view of the liquor store and the service station. Each room sounds different, smells different, and feels different. I used to arrive at check-in filled with uncertainty, because every new room was so disorienting.

"I just want to know how to get to the toilet in the dark" was how I explained my desperation to the front-desk clerk. "I want to be able to navigate the room without hitting a wall or the doorjamb or a cupboard. Please! If I'm always in the same room, I can wake up in the morning and know which side of the bed I'm on."

So room 4 has become my room. I know its nooks and crannies, where the electrical outlets are, and that I have to turn the showerhead toward the wall to avoid flooding the bathroom floor. I know to pull the battery out of the clock because its tick is too loud. I know where the blankets are when it gets cold, and I barely notice the passing trains and the shaking fridge. When I first arrive, I know to adjust the blinds and tuck in the edges of the curtains to block the streetlight, and I know to open the windows to let out the smell of cleaning products. I know not to overfill the kettle (because it splatters boiling water onto the counter) and to turn on the table lamps (because the overhead fluorescents glare too brightly), and I know the roles of all five remotes. It took me some time to get to know room 4, but now that I do, I sleep like a log—and in the middle of the night, I can get up and walk to the toilet in the pitch-black.

So there's the truth about me. I like to think of myself as spontaneous, as footloose and fancy-free. I'm a person who believes that getting lost is part of the adventure and who's willing to hang-glide off a cliff on short notice. But I actually love consistency. I love routine and rituals. I won't turn around on a walk without touching a rock or a tree. When I go into the ocean at the end of my street, I don't count it as a real swim unless I put my head under the water three times. Any less than that is just a dip. I've used the exact same shampoo and conditioner for years, I always buy the same brand of Jarlsberg cheese, and I like to drink the same wine. And when one of these brands isn't available, I'm not a happy camper.

My love of sameness is just how my brain is wired. But instead of chastising myself, I've learned that these habits are just a beautiful component of what makes me *me*. We all have our quirks, and these characteristics are created by how we think, sense, and feel.

The ways that we interpret information, process sensory input, and experience emotion are as diverse as we are. When I was a child, I was told, "Every person is unique." I thought of this as meaning "I have freckles and you don't" or "I have hazel eyes and you have blue." But over the course of my life, I've come to understand that this uniqueness relates to how our brains work. Autistic and neurodivergent people are wired differently from neurotypical people, and in these differences lie many lessons about how our perceptions and views of the world are constructed.

Who you are is shaped by your thoughts. I'm an overthinker and will try to look at situations and experiences from every angle. I turn them around and around in my head, and these thoughts can keep me up at night. I'm easily distracted, and because of this I constantly lose things and leave my belongings on buses, in taxis, and at café tables.

I'm also highly emotional. I cry all the time, and tears come easily. I cry when I'm sad, happy, frustrated, or angry. I cry when I watch movies and read books. I cry when people tell me stories of their hurt, but also when they share their successes. My tears flow when I see another person's tears, even if I don't know why they're crying. I cry so much that once, as a child, I was removed from a movie theater because I couldn't stop sobbing when Bambi's mother died. (Sorry for the spoiler.)

I'm super-conscious of my senses. I love the way they all work together to take in the world. I like to listen with my eyes closed and break down what I hear: leaves rustling, a bird's song, the footsteps on the floor above me. I love the sounds of snorkeling—the tinkle, crack, and click. I have a fondness for soft light. My favorite time of day is the gloaming, that light just before sunset when shadows are long and everything is golden. And I can't live without the feel of water on my skin—baths, oceans, lakes, or just splashing it on my face.

In the ways you and I perceive the world, we might be as different as day and night. But we also have the chance to appreciate these incredible differences in how others think and sense and feel. It's in these differences that we're given the most wonderful opportunity to view life through a whole new lens. If we think about the vastness of this—that every single human being is having their own experience and that our own perspective is just ours—it makes learning about one another an endless journey of discovery.

# 1

# Emily's Diapers

The Martins lived in a suburban cul-de-sac surrounded by cookie-cutter houses. The interior of their house was a jolting combination of mission-brown walls and orange laminate countertops, and the only heater was in the living room, which consequently became the hub of activity. And there was always a lot of activity. Leslie had three beautiful children under seven; the youngest had been born a few weeks before, and her two older kids were autistic. Leslie's partner worked as a long-haul trucker during the week and came home only on weekends, which meant Leslie was the sole parent five days a week.

This was quite different from the house I was living in with a bunch of students at the time. It was a typical student house; there were always dishes in the sink, trash that didn't quite make it to the curb, and constant arguments over who had eaten whose food. While living there, I was studying education at university and had a part-time job as a community support worker for people with disabilities. It was a perfect job for me, as it allowed me to get the kind of hands-on experience you couldn't get at school. As a young woman without children, I didn't understand the reality of families with young kids, much less families with children with disabilities. This job connected theory and real-life experience for me.

The Martins were a loving family who were grateful for my help, and they always welcomed me into their home with open arms. I was an extra pair of hands, and I'd do whatever they needed me to do. On the days I worked, I'd arrive at six a.m. to help get the kids ready for school, then I'd come back in the afternoon for after-school activities and move into the busy hours of bath, dinner, and bedtime stories. I became a part of the family.

The late afternoon, just before dinner, is, as all parents of young children know, the witching hour when chaos rules the house. As it approaches, it can fill parents with dread. After a long day when all they hope for is calm, parents find themselves in a quagmire created by overstimulated children and their own exhaustion, and the whimpering, whining, clinging, and general malaise can rapidly escalate into tantrums and tears. Time slows down, making the witching hour feel like it's days long.

One afternoon, everyone, including Leslie, was tired and hungry. The kids needed to be bathed and fed, but then disaster struck: Leslie ran out of diapers, not only for the baby but also for the other two children, who were not yet toilet-trained.

"Jodi, could you do a run to the supermarket for me?" Leslie asked over the heads of three kids and a mountain of laundry. "We need pull-ups, extra-large, and newborn."

"No worries," I said. To relieve some of Leslie's stress, I suggested I take Emily, the eldest of the three kids.

Emily was a curious and busy six-year-old who always looked like she'd spent the day in the wild; she was rumpled and scruffy and usually covered in dirt and grime. Emily's giggle was infectious; she was caught in her own world, laughing out loud at things unseen by the rest of us. Her high-pitched chuckle brought a smile to my face every time I heard it. Emily was able to communicate her day-to-day wants and needs as well as label objects, follow simple instructions, and make requests, but she didn't have the speech to communicate the things that brought her happiness or pain.

When we arrived at the supermarket, the parking lot was relatively full; people were doing their after-work shopping. I'd been there with Leslie and the children on many occasions. It was a well-known nationwide chain; if you were familiar with one, chances are you could navigate them all. Leslie had taught me how to engage the children in the process of shopping. Her strategy was to give the two older kids pictures of what was on her shopping list and take them down each aisle, explaining what was needed in that aisle from the list. Leslie had created a route that was familiar to the kids; she always began in one specific aisle and finished in another. In this way, she broke down the supermarket into small parts.

*I've got this*, I thought. I'd seen Leslie do it a dozen times. I knew this space well, and I believed I would be returning to Leslie as the triumphant diaper deliverer—but not everything turns out the way we plan.

We all know our own supermarket well. We know exactly what aisle we need to travel to grab an item, exactly where the product is in that aisle, and which route to take through the store to quickly tick items off our shopping list.

But think about when you have to shop at a *new* supermarket. Perhaps you're on vacation in a different town or you need to pick up something for dinner when you're coming home from the other side of the city. Why is the milk not next to the butter? Who on earth stocks the canned tuna next to tea and coffee? Everything is different—and annoying.

Or maybe your local supermarket had an upgrade. Management changed the layout of the aisles to boost sales, or they decided to stock new brands and discontinue others. That sense of familiarity you had when you first walked in quickly fades because the mental systems and structure you've created have been broken. You'll feel a little agitated and frustrated at first, but you'll work it out after a few visits, and then that configuration becomes your new normal. It's a small change in a routine that can send even the most adaptable of us into a tailspin.

Most people have difficulty with change, particularly if the change is sudden. We like to know what is happening next and how it will look and what to expect. We are creatures of habit, and by following the same route or completing a task in the same way every time, we are rewarded with a feeling of calmness and safety. We love things to be simple and easy.

It's hard to learn a new skill or develop a new habit. The human brain is a complicated structure full of billions of cells that need to work together in order to sense, emote, and react. They control every aspect of your life, including your thoughts, memories, emotions, heartbeat, and breath. Brain cells communicate via neurons. These neurons find the most efficient path to convey their messages, and when they've traveled this route a few times, it becomes the preferred way.

Learning a new skill, like swimming or riding a bike, challenges neural pathways. It's not until you have repeated a particular action numerous times that it becomes second nature. Once these pathways are embedded in your brain, you don't need to think *How do I swim?* or *How do I ride a bike?* You just do it, on autopilot.

When we come across something new and different, our brains must create new paths, and this can be difficult and complex. It's like walking a track through wilderness you've never visited before: You have to navigate the terrain, weave through trees and climb over boulders, all while not being sure of where you're going. You must pay attention to make sure you don't trip or get lost, and it can be exhausting.

Next time you pass through this wilderness, though, it will be more familiar. You'll take the easiest route over and over until you've created a well-trodden, well-loved path. Your neurons create paths like this that you stick to because they're easier and take far less energy to navigate than new ones. The more you do something, the more it becomes a habit. The downside is that sometimes the unexpected happens, and you can't remain on autopilot. When things change, you have to change too. But this is much harder for some people than it is for others.

When there is a sudden change in our lives, we must use all our flexible thinking to manage it. Cognitive flexibility takes place in the frontal lobe of the brain, which sits just above the eyes. This part of the brain synchronizes all higher-level brain activity; it's where thinking, decision-making, and problem-solving takes place.

Being adaptive, flexible, and able to shift your thoughts quickly is a high-level skill. The brain interprets sudden change as a warning and sends your body into protective mode. The process evolved to warn humans about saber-toothed tigers but now it kicks in when your computer crashes . . . or when the supermarket layout changes.

Neurotypical people take for granted the ability to shift their thoughts. For many autistic people, rigid or repetitive thinking is a component of their neurological system. The need for sameness is central to an autistic person's way of moving through the world, making it even harder to adapt to change.

Autistic people can be highly sensitive when it comes to changes in their environment, structure, or routine. New situations, the unfamiliar, and the element of surprise can be difficult to navigate.

When Emily and I entered the supermarket that afternoon, *everything* had changed. The supermarket had had a makeover, and the aisles had all shifted from one place to another. Nothing made sense anymore. Not to me, and certainly not to Emily.

Her meltdown started before we even got to the first aisle. Emily demonstrated her displeasure by grinding her teeth, which was an early warning sign of things to come.

"I know, I know, it's all wrong," I said to Emily. To try to distract her and keep her from becoming overwhelmed, I gave her a picture of the diapers. But then I realized that I didn't know where the diapers were. What aisle were they in now?

This should have been so simple: find the diapers and get out. But the layout was all wrong. Where was the first aisle, the one that started with the deli and moved to the vegetables? Then the next aisle with bread and cereal, tea and coffee and long-life milk, and the one after that, with the pasta and noodles? The first aisle now had a bakery and health foods, and there were wide-open spaces in the middle of the store.

Not only that, but when I looked at the signs above the aisles for help, I realized they had yet to be changed. The sign above what was now the rice aisle read CANNED VEGETABLES, and the sign reading CHIPS AND CHOCOLATE was above an aisle full of cereal. So even the visual indicators of how it was all supposed to work were wrong.

"Come on, Em," I said. "Let's just find the diapers."

But Emily was having none of it. In seconds, her emotions went from 0 to 100, like a Ferrari. Her teeth-grinding spiraled into short sharp screeches, and before I could blink an eye, she turned and ran. Emily let me know that the supermarket was wrong by darting away like a frightened deer, quick and agile. I chased after her.

And then I couldn't find her. I couldn't find Emily.

The diapers ceased to exist, as did the shelves and the people and the cans and the boxes. I had only one job: *find Emily*.

After a few anxious moments, my heart pounding, I heard her. Emily was pulling things from the shelves and throwing them onto the ground. And she was yelling. Screaming. By the time I reached her, she couldn't hear me. She could no longer settle herself or trust that I wasn't part of this change. She cried and beat her arms and legs. I stood over her and tried to keep the groceries from being ripped off the shelves, but people were gathering and Emily was not calming. Everyone stopped and stared, and I just wanted to protect her. So I picked her up.

I knew it wasn't the right thing to do. People in the midst of a meltdown might not respond well when someone lays hands on them. In fact, it can kick their bodies into overdrive and often makes it worse. I knew this was true for Emily; I knew it was wrong to pick her up, but I did it anyway because I needed to get us out of there. It was no longer a safe space for either of us.

Emily thrashed and kicked and screamed blue murder. I hated myself for having done this to her. She kept struggling as I took her out of the supermarket and into the parking lot. I finally got her to the car, but now I had to strap her into the child seat. I *had* to, because that was the law, and I needed to get her home.

But Emily was in survival mode. She threw out her arms and legs and arched her back, pushing me and everything else away. No matter how hard I tried, I couldn't get her into that seat. I couldn't because *she* couldn't let me. Emily flung her arms out and smacked me in the face. She hit me hard on the bridge of my nose. Now there were tears in my eyes for many reasons.

"*Why don't you control your child!*" snarled a woman on her way into the supermarket.

*Why. Don't. You. Control. Your. Child.*

My internal response: *Fuck you.*

*Fuck you and your Victorian attitude that children should be seen and not heard. Fuck you that you think any human should be controlled. Fuck you that you think that parenting is about control. Fuck you and your judgment. Fuck you that you can see another woman struggling and not give her a hand. Fuck you that you are not helping. Fuck you. Fuck you. Fuck you.*

"She's autistic" is what came out of my mouth. "Please understand!" I felt like shouting.

It crushed me that I felt the need to explain Emily's behavior to a complete stranger, especially one who lacked caring and sympathy. Autism should never be something you apologize for—in fact, this stranger should have been apologizing to *us*.

I sat on the edge of the back seat, legs dangling out of the door, and stopped trying to get Emily into the car seat. I stopped thinking that I needed to calm her pain. I stopped hushing her and trying to make her behavior fit others' expectations of what was "correct" for a child. I just sat.

Emily's screams slowly turned to sobs and then whimpers. As I sat, I was acutely aware that, while I'd done this once, her mom must have experienced this multiple times—and while juggling two other children. Leslie would have been judged by strangers, would have had people stare at her and her family and make assumptions about her fitness as a mother. Leslie had no doubt felt the need, time and time again, to "explain" her daughter's differences. My heart hurt thinking that she had to do this. My heart hurt that maybe no one had ever reached out to help her.

At that moment, I made a promise to myself: whenever I saw a person struggling with a child, I would offer help or a word of encouragement. Sometimes all of us need a little help. We all need a little kindness.

Then I considered that passing stranger. She would soon experience the frustration of the changed supermarket. She wouldn't suffer as Emily had, but she too would struggle.

We all react differently to the unexpected and unplanned, but most people find it difficult. Some will be quick to adapt; some will swear under their breath; some will have a rant; and some will experience panic and confusion. Next time you see someone having an emotional reaction to a sudden change, be compassionate and understand it's just the person's brain saying, *Why can't we keep it simple?*

# 2

# Eric's Bowl

Eric dressed like an old man, even though he was in his thirties. He loved to wear Velcro sandals with socks and sweater-vests over plain cotton T-shirts. He had an assortment of cargo shorts and filled the pockets with useful items, which meant he was never without a hankie or a pencil stub. Eric had many favorite things, including his rectangular-head toothbrush (he had no time for diamond-head ones), his favorite towel (a bath towel at the perfect size of fifty-five by twenty-seven inches), and his favorite bowl.

And Eric's bowl was broken.

When I met Eric, he lived in a residential setting with four housemates who all had intellectual disabilities. At that time, I was working as part of a multidisciplinary team of speech therapists, occupational therapists, psychologists, and educators who specialized in autism, and we provided support and education to the wider community. I was the one who received the confused phone call from a staff member who was with Eric in his home.

"His bowl is broken," the disability support worker said. "But I don't understand what the problem is. There are plenty of other bowls in the house."

But there were no other "favorite" bowls, and Eric was not happy. He yelled and swore and vowed that he would never eat breakfast again. And he didn't—not for weeks.

This might not seem like a big deal; a lot of us skip the first meal of the day, and Eric was still eating lunch and dinner. But he had an anti-seizure medication that needed to be taken first thing in the morning with food. Eric had epilepsy, and missing his pills put him at high risk of having a tonic-clonic (grand mal) seizure. For Eric, his favorite bowl and these pills went together as part of the same breakfast system. And now that the system had collapsed, Eric was in danger of collapsing along with it.

We all have our favorite things. Some people like to drink tea from a chunky mug, others from a china cup with a thin, delicate rim. Some people love scratchy towels and others soft, snuggly ones. Some prefer stemless wineglasses and for others, the stem is the most important part of the wine-drinking experience. We have our favorite things, but most of the time we never wonder why. With a little self-examination, we might discover that we love certain objects because they have become part of our system.

All of us create systems, whether it's the way we arrange our homes or how we complete specific tasks, and a lot of our systems can appear somewhat the same. This is why you can usually navigate around another person's home—because of the similarities in how people organize space. (It's almost an unwritten rule that the top drawer is for cutlery, the second for utensils, the third for foil, and the bottom for tea towels.) But many systems differ. It might be a specific way of organizing the linen closet—some people fold their towels and sheets, and others roll them. People might hang clothes on the line or rack differently; some might peg similar clothing in the same row—underwear lined up together and socks hung in pairs—while others might arrange by color or household member. Even the smallest tasks of the day have a system, like the way to make a cup of tea. Water, tea bag, then milk? Or milk, water, then tea bag? (This is a hotly debated issue in Commonwealth countries.)

Systems are the basis of routines, a kind of procedural manual to follow when performing activities or tasks. Sometimes it can be difficult to identify why you've established these systems. They may come from your parents or the way you were taught to do something as a child. Maybe you prefer a system for practical reasons that override aesthetics, like leaving the dishes to air-dry on the rack rather than hand-drying them and immediately putting them away. Or maybe you prefer to give up practicality in favor of the look and feel—just how many pillows do you have on your bed right now, and how are they arranged? Once you have found a specific system that suits you, your brain clings to it.

Have you ever moved in with someone and had a clash of systems? It happens! It would be so easy if everyone shared the same systems—if your housemate stacked the dishwasher the way you wanted it stacked or your partner made the bed the way you wanted it made, right? When people do it "your" way, you remain calm and relaxed—everything is as it should be. But if someone interrupts your process or changes your method, you can become irritated.

I have a system for vegetables. When cooking, I like to have vegetables cut into certain shapes, widths, and lengths. Carrots that are going into a wok will be julienned, and those that are being thrown into a casserole will be cut into rounds. I have this system because I want things to look a certain way when the meal is complete. (I'm a person who goes through cookbooks just to look at the pictures.) My vegetable system isn't a big deal if I'm alone in the kitchen, but when someone casually asks if I want help with the chopping, my heart rate increases and I become a little anxious. No, I don't want someone in *my* kitchen not following *my* vegetable system! Luckily, I have the communication skills to express this need. If I must let someone into my kitchen, I can demonstrate exactly how I want the vegetables cut and even provide a visual aid by chopping a few myself so my expectations can be met.

Not everyone has the capacity to communicate their system, however, no matter how important it is to them. For some autistic people, it's a struggle to explain why certain things need to be done in certain ways. This is heightened by the fact that while neurotypical people like systems, some autistic people *love* them.

Many autistic people love patterns in their everyday lives. A pattern can be easily followed because it's all about repetition—just ask any knitter or quilter. Patterns help us to understand sequence, they're predictable, and they follow logic. For some autistic people, the systems of daily tasks create patterns that can be easily understood and then replicated. It keeps things simple. The challenge comes when there is a random change or shift, and the pattern no longer follows its regular step-by-step progression.

Many neurotypical people don't understand why something as simple as switching breakfast bowls causes so much anxiety and anguish, but there are always reasons why autistic people do the things they do. If you take the time to try to understand why someone has created the system, it will more than likely make complete sense. You might even find the system brilliant.

The first step is not to make assumptions about what someone wants and needs or why their system is important to them. The first step is to ask why this specific system is so essential.

"Why is the bowl so important to you?" I asked Eric.

Every morning of Eric's life, he has had two Weet-Bix for breakfast. These are thin, rectangular biscuits of shredded wheat, about four inches by two inches. To most people, they're just ordinary breakfast. But to Eric, there is no more perfect breakfast than two Weet-Bix with milk and honey.

"There is good nutritional value in Weet-Bix," Eric told me. He then listed by heart all the ingredients to back up this fact. Whole-grain cereals, such as wheat, rye, sorghum, oats, and rice; sugar—"which is good in small doses," he assured me—along with puffed wheat, barley malt extract, coconut, salt, honey, vegetable oil, and the vitamins thiamine, riboflavin, niacin, vitamin E, and iron.

"There's also the terrible possibility that if Weet-Bix are mistreated," he continued, "they'll become soggy. And when Weet-Bix are soggy, they are porridge. And who would want to eat soggy food, let alone porridge?"

There was no way that Eric was eating soggy anything. Through trial and error over the course of years, Eric had developed a Weet-Bix system that was an engineering feat. Two Weet-Bix are placed side by side in the bowl. ("One Weet-Bix is not enough," he told me, "and three is too many.") There must, however, be a gap between them of at least a quarter of an inch. The Weet-Bix must not be broken—they must be whole; two half Weet-Bix does not equal one whole Weet-Bix.

Once the Weet-Bix are in position, the correct amount of the correct type of honey (not creamed, *never* creamed) is drizzled along each Weet-Bix. Measure this with a teaspoon: one teaspoon of honey per Weet-Bix.

The correct amount of milk is then added (two-thirds of a cup, precisely measured, and always full-fat, never *ever* skim milk). The milk should be poured directly into the bowl, around the two Weet-Bix and in the gap between them (never *ever* on top of the Weet-Bix).

Voilà! The milk is absorbed into the Weet-Bix from the bottom but does not touch the top or interfere with the consistency of the honey. It soaks through just enough so that you don't end up with dry shredded wheat stuck to the roof of your mouth, but the crispy upper layer still gives you some crunch. To Eric, this was the only way to eat Weet-Bix. The correct way.

"And Eric, the bowl?"

"That bowl was the *perfect* Weet-Bix bowl," Eric said. He showed me the broken bowl. When it was whole, all the edges were the same height, jutting up at right angles from the base, so the milk absorbed at exactly the same rate. The bowl was wide enough to fit the two Weet-Bix in perfect symmetry with exactly the right amount of space in between them for milk.

It made complete sense. This bowl would never work:

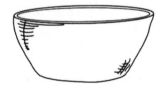

And neither would this one:

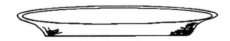

Only Eric's bowl would work. We just needed to find another bowl like Eric's.

Thanks to the internet, we began a worldwide search for the perfect replacement Weet-Bix bowl. Eric and I lost ourselves in search engines and scoured every kitchen site we could find.

Finally, there it was: the perfect Weet-Bix bowl, take two.

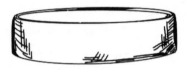

Eric was thrilled when his new bowl arrived. The next morning, the bowl, Weet-Bix box, honey, milk, jug, and measuring spoons were quickly lined up on the kitchen counter, along with his medication. Now that Eric's system was complete, he sat and ate the perfect, well-organized cereal with relish.

If you look at the world from only your own perspective, another person's system might make little sense—or no sense at all. But when I saw the world from Eric's point of view, his insistence that without his bowl, he would never eat breakfast again was completely understandable. Eric and his perfect Weet-Bix system just required the right bowl.

So next time you drink your tea from *your* mug or reach into the cupboard and choose *your* favorite towel (either rolled or folded) or you take down *your* favorite wineglass and pour yourself a glass of *your* favorite wine, ask yourself: *Why is this my favorite? Why do I like this one so much? Is it part of my system?*

# 3

# Sebastian's Spider-Man

Sebastian's whole world was Spider-Man. His room was filled with all things Spidey. His bedcover and pillows were decorated with webs, and his walls were plastered in Spidey posters. He had Spider-Man DVDs, figurines, comic books, and Legos. He knew all the incarnations of Spider-Man from the movies, and given that he was only six, this was impressive. He was into the Spider-Man of Tobey Maguire, Andrew Garfield, Tom Holland, and even Shinji Todo, the Japanese Spider-Man.

Sebastian was very determined and his enthusiasm was contagious. He loved to chat and could talk up a storm, engaging everyone in conversation—as long as that conversation was about Spidey! Sebastian lived in his own Spider-Man fantasy realm, but not everyone loved Spider-Man as much as he did. The staffers at Sebastian's school, for example, were not part of the Spider-Man fan club.

I visited the school early one morning to discuss how best to support Sebastian. In a classroom with a colorful array of striped mats and cushions on the floor and kids' paintings of rainbows, crooked houses, and smiling yellow suns on the walls, the staff and I sat on tiny chairs with our legs splayed to the side.

"He's a delightful kid," one staff member said, "full of bounce and energy. But we've had some problems over the last few months."

Another teacher told me that Sebastian's Spider-Man obsession had become a "real issue." Sebastian wouldn't participate in any activities unless they had to do with Spider-Man. He wouldn't do any part of the set curriculum, not the reading or the math.

The school had asked Sebastian's mom to keep all his Spider-Man paraphernalia out of the classroom. They asked that he not wear his Spidey T-shirts, carry his Spidey backpack, or bring his Spidey lunch box. And he was *definitely* not to bring any Spidey figurines to school. "Sebastian's infatuation needed to be stopped, as it was hindering his development," the teacher said.

*And this could hinder his happiness*, I thought.

I decided to observe Sebastian in class to see how he was coping without his Spidey stuff. He entered the classroom wearing jeans and a cardigan. His short brown hair was parted on the side and slicked down with water, though wild tufts stood out at every angle in the back. He was quieter than I'd ever seen him. He did his worksheets at the table, sat on the floor with the rest of the class for story time, and ate lunch from his nondescript blue lunch box. But he wasn't present. He was constantly mouthing words silently to himself and calling his classmates Aunt May or Betty and his teachers Doc Ock.

I was watching him move through his morning out of the corner of my eye—and then I saw it! Under the desk, Sebastian turned his hand, extended his arm, and touched two fingers to the middle of his palm, and an imaginary web shot out of his wrist.

"Who are you? What's your name?" I asked him later that day.

"Peter," he quietly stated. "Peter Parker."

\*   \*   \*

You can't take away an interest. You can take away everything that is related to the interest, but that has never stopped anyone from thinking about the things they love. Just as Peter Parker could not reveal his identity as Spider-Man, Sebastian hid his fixation on his favorite superhero by wearing civilian clothing. But this didn't take away his passion.

Many young children have an interest that fascinates them, and about a third of all kids between two and six years old will become fixated on a topic at some point. I have a niece who thought she was a fairy and wore the same fairy dress night and day until she was five. Hordes of children will watch garbage trucks on collection day or bulldozers on construction sites. And as most of us know, dinosaurs are definitely not extinct in many kids' imaginations.

Generally, once neurotypical children reach school age, their fascination with any one specific area fades. As kids develop peer relationships, their interests expand, and they will follow the fads of their friends. I remember wanting a yo-yo because *everyone* had a yo-yo, a mood ring because *everyone* had a mood ring, and roller skates because—you guessed it. As I grew up, I lost interest in these things, but for many autistic kids, their special interests do not shift as quickly as those of the neurotypical kids around them.

When my nephew was younger, he knew the names and jersey numbers of all the football players in our Australian Football League. He knew all of their statistics: "He's one hundred kilos and one-point-nine-one meters tall," he'd tell me about a particular player before moving on to how many games he'd played in his career. He could tell you the name of every team that had won the grand final for the past hundred years and how far the average player ran in one game (8.7 miles, if you are wondering).

My nephew is now sixteen and still knows a lot of football stats. And while he has grown and developed in a typical way and his interests have broadened, he remains dedicated to his footie team. In fact, my whole extended family follows the same team, and this collective passion binds us, at least in the winter months when they're playing. It's great to have interests and even better when you can share your enthusiasm with others.

One of the greatest joys of spending thirty years working with neurodivergent people has been learning so much about their wonderful and diverse special interests. One of my clients could look at a map of Australia and point to any town, national park, desert, or river you named in milliseconds. Another could tell you the day of your birth if you gave him the date and the year. I loved one woman who could name all three hundred (and counting) dog breeds, tell me every breed's history, and give me the pros and cons of each.

I've spent time learning the ins and outs of Star Trek, Star Wars, Pokémon, and K-pop; I now know a bit about the World Wrestling Federation, Academy Award winners in costume design, and Hello Kitty. And the detail of my clients' knowledge is always startling. Years ago, I mentioned to someone that I was going to plant some vegetables on the weekend. I was given a full rundown on permaculture—its history, design principles, zones, and companion planting. To this day I still plant marigolds with my tomatoes and alyssum with my lettuce. Many neurodivergent people could earn PhDs for the vast knowledge they have in their favorite subject areas.

You get to witness pure joy when an autistic person raves about a passion. But for many neurodivergent people, it's not just that they *want* to talk about their passion—they *need* to talk about it. It's a component of their neurologic system.

For autistic people, interests are not just hobbies; they are central to their well-being. Sometimes called obsessions or restricted, circumscribed, or specialized interests, these intense passions are a core and extremely common aspect of autism. Many special interests involve gathering facts, collecting objects, and cataloging them into systems. This establishes familiar structure, order, and certainty—all qualities that an autistic brain loves. For some people, sharing their interests with others provides the extrinsic reward of social interaction, but for many autistic people, pursuing their special interest is intrinsically motivating. The reward comes from engaging in the interest itself.

Jamie, for example, loved locks. All kinds of locks. He loved padlocks, knob locks, cam locks, rim locks...every type. He loved really old locks and would spend hours shopping for antique locks online. Jamie had studied the mechanics of lock systems; he'd bought a key cutter and taught himself to make keys. He had a particular passion for old rusty locks that had no keys, and he would spend days on end making keys so they could be opened. At twenty-one years old, he was a master locksmith without a locksmith job; he could have been a pro at breaking and entering, but he had no desire for anything behind the door. He was only interested in the lock itself.

This incredible capacity to hyper-focus is a characteristic of autism. Autistic people can concentrate on one activity or topic to the exclusion of everything else. Some people are so hyper-focused when researching or engaging in their interests that they forget to eat, drink, and sleep.

I sometimes think that if I had this level of hyper-focus, I could have been a great scientist. When I was in high school, we sat in the science lab at high wooden tables studded with Bunsen burners. In every lesson, I sat against the same wall with three classmates sitting to my right. On the wall to my left was a huge poster of the periodic table of the elements. That table's wonderful system fascinated me. The poster told me a story about all the elements and their electrons. It told me about atoms and the protons in their nuclei. The elements had numbers and nicknames. Some of those nicknames were logical, like H for hydrogen; others were not so logical, like Fe for iron and Au for gold (although, as an Australian, I have always remembered this every Olympics).

I loved that periodic table. At the beginning of class, I would look at it and try hard to memorize all those letters, then link the letters to the numbers and the numbers to the colors. It was confusing, yet beautiful.

But for me, humans always get in the way, and Sam was one of those humans. The periodic table was to my left, and Sam was to my right. All that separated Sam and me was a Bunsen burner.

I was fourteen, and Sam distracted me in every science class. Sam smelled of sweat and boy deodorant. He had curly dirty blond hair and a loud cheeky laugh. He didn't know the periodic table of elements existed. And when I sat next to Sam, neither did I.

When Sam was there, my body twisted and oriented toward him; my gaze was always directed to the right. When Sam said my name, I couldn't react fast enough. When Sam spoke to me, I nodded. I nodded *a lot*. When Sam laughed, I laughed. When Sam leaned toward me, I leaned toward him. And the periodic table of the elements to the left? It never stood a chance! My highly distracted, socially motivated brain (and teenage hormones) got in the way of my future as a brilliant chemist.

I'm not alone in this. As most young people grow, they care more and more about other people and want to be part of the gang. High school is a social experiment for all of us, but in a world where social interaction is confusing, people are complex, and the senses are overwhelmed, a special interest can create calm and relieve stress.

I'm well aware of the difficulties that many autistic people can have in forming and maintaining relationships. I know that navigating the world of social nuance can be complex, and meeting someone for the first time can be difficult. I also know that when someone talks about their interests, it gives them a chance to shine. When I meet a new client, if we're into the same thing, brilliant; if not, I make sure that our first interactions are built around their passion, then I learn as much about it as I possibly can. Talking with people about their interests builds rapport, and common interests form a foundation for wonderful friendships. With clients, I always make their interests the basis of our relationship.

Ethan was one of these clients.

Ethan was into motorbikes. Before I met him, I'd read his referral form, which asks about a person's interests. Ethan had completed his own form and he had provided so much detail about motorbikes that it filled every line and every margin and the other side of the page.

He arrived for our first appointment wearing his motorbike leathers and carrying a helmet. He was an imposing figure and took up most of the doorframe before he entered the room, but his size did not match how gently he walked or how much consideration he gave to deciding where he wanted to sit. He was so soft-spoken that I had trouble hearing him, and he responded to my questions with monosyllables.

And then he saw it: the motorbike magazine. Before he arrived, I had run out and bought *Cycle World*. I'd placed it on the coffee table, not in full view but visible among the other magazines.

Ethan picked it up and he was off, telling me about Yamahas, Suzukis, Ducatis, Kawasakis, and HOGs. He talked excitedly about MotoGP, where the top speed was recorded at 226 miles per hour and the tires of the bikes are warmed to 194 degrees before the race. He listed some of his heroes: Valentino Rossi and Marc Márquez and Mick Doohan. Then his checkered flag came down briefly and he asked, "Do you ride motorbikes?"

"Only in Southeast Asia," I replied. "And I do have a massive scar on my knee from coming off one when I was nineteen!"

Ethan pulled back the sleeve of his leather jacket and showed me a huge and nasty scar running across his elbow. And then our conversation broadened. What had started with motorbikes led to one story after another of our injuries and accidents. Our scars opened the door to talking about our lives and our pasts. When Ethan left that day, he said he would bring me a couple more magazines for my "collection."

We all appreciate it when someone asks about our interests. We love sharing information and having people genuinely listen to what we have to say. I adore the term *info-dumping*, meaning when someone gives you a large volume of information about their interest. When someone is info-dumping, I listen hard and think about when and where I might be able to use all this knowledge. (Definitely at pub trivia.)

Some autistic people have special interests that last a lifetime; others drop their previous interests as soon as new interests are discovered. Some special interests are sparked not by curiosity but by fear. I knew an autistic child who, fearful of storms, became an expert in meteorology, and another who, scared of spiders, became an arachnologist in order to understand and allay their fear. As people say, "Knowledge is power."

Kyle was one of those kids whose interest is motivated by

fear. He was a serious child who read early and read a lot. He loved books, TV, and movies, particularly Pixar movies. Kyle would sit as close to the TV screen as he could, turn out the lights, and create his own front-row seat in the cinema.

When Kyle was five years old, *Finding Nemo* came out. It's a beautiful movie with gorgeous underwater scenes and hilarious characters. While most kids watched the whole thing multiple times, Kyle watched just one scene over and over. With his hand glued to the remote, he would rewind, play, rewind, play, rewind—but just the opening scene. At the drop-off where the sanctuary of the coral reef disappears into the deep ocean, Marlin (Nemo's dad) is attacked and knocked unconscious, and Coral (Nemo's mom) and almost all of her clownfish eggs—except the one that Nemo later hatches from—are eaten by a massive, sharp-fanged barracuda. It's the first moment of the movie, and for Kyle it was traumatizing.

Kyle was transfixed and terrified by this scene. He would talk nonstop about barracudas, ask lots of questions about them. He drew and painted barracudas and he read about them. This fixation may have driven some people mad—there are only so many barracuda facts you need—but Kyle's parents took it on with relish and helped shape Kyle's future. They broadened his interest by buying him books on ocean predators and asking him questions about sharks, moray eels, orcas, and lionfish. They gave him a season pass to the aquarium for his birthday, which heightened his fascination with all marine life.

Kyle never lost interest. As a teenager he got a job at the aquarium and went on to study marine biology at university. He is currently researching plankton, "the basis of all marine ecosystems and responsible for our survival as humans," he told me. I have no doubt that Kyle will research his way into saving the oceans and the air we breathe. Thank you, Nemo.

Not all special interests are as wonderful as marine life. Sometimes autistic people get hooked on an interest that can be harmful or even illegal, and then they need support to be guided to interests that are safer for them. But the majority of autistic people's interests are captivating and fun and support their mental health, and, as they did for Kyle, they can lead to fascinating professions.

We all want to follow pursuits that fill us with enthusiasm. Passion is not about having extensive knowledge; it's a feeling. It gives us purpose. It fills us with joy and gives life meaning. When we are passionate *about something*, we are happier.

Sebastian ticked the boxes on his worksheets, colored between the lines, and sat among his peers on the bright mat, but he was a shadow of his old self. He was going through the motions without any excitement or eagerness. He was no longer a sprightly, chatty little boy but one who spoke quietly to himself under his breath. There was no bounce or energy anymore. He was just sad. Sebastian was missing the love of his life—he was missing Spidey.

And watching this enthusiastic boy disengage was so concerning to the staff that they decided it was time for Spider-Man's return.

Sebastian's teachers adjusted the curriculum for him and worked Spidey into his learning. He counted spiderwebs for math, learned to write and read words with Spider-Man themes, and presented facts on spiders for show-and-tell. He was sent on "missions" to help pack up toys and sharpen pencils and wash the paintbrushes and water the plants. He thrived.

"We went one step further," the teachers told me later that same year. "With Great Power Comes Great Responsibility" became the class motto.

# 4

# Heidi's Bed

Heidi was quite alone in the world. She had moved to Australia from Canada and was estranged from her family. She went to work each day in a large distribution warehouse but had no work friends and didn't spend time with people outside of her job. She wore glasses that were too big for her, so she constantly pushed them up the bridge of her nose. And the only splash of color she ever wore came from one of an array of silky scarves that she wrapped around her black outfits. Winter, summer, spring, fall—always black.

There was a rental crisis in the area where Heidi lived, and when the lease on the apartment she had called home for the past three years ended, she had to find a new place...in two days. Her search was complicated by the fact that she needed to live on her own. She refused to live with others. She'd tried it before, and it had ended in arguments and tears. She was searching for a one-person haven from the chaotic world, but until she found it, she needed somewhere to stay, and she needed it fast.

"There's no way that I'm sleeping in a bed in a hotel," Heidi told me. "I would rather sleep in my car than stay there!"

"Oh, Heidi. It'll be really clean. The sheets are changed every day; you don't have to worry."

"It's not that," she responded. "I could never sleep thinking of all the bad people who may have slept in the bed or the bad things that may have happened to it. I would be so sad for the bed and what it must be feeling."

*Feeling? What do you mean, the bed has feelings?*

My brother's family are like the Weasleys in Harry Potter. Their home is full of laughter and love, but it's slightly shambolic and everything is used by everyone. You can be almost certain that any towel in the bathroom has been used to wipe several people's faces and bums. The one bathroom that they all share (which also has the washing machine in it) has a cup on the sink with more toothbrushes in it than members of the household.

"Which toothbrush is yours?" I once asked my niece as we stood side by side about to brush.

"I've no idea. I just grab one," she said, shoving a toothbrush with bent bristles into her mouth. This comment would turn the stomach of any dental hygienist.

We all have objects that we think should be ours and ours alone. In every school and organization I have ever worked in, you brought in your own coffee mug to distinguish it from the communal-use mugs. The cupboards in these places were filled with cups for visitors, and most people got slightly put out when they saw "their" mugs (labeled BEST MOM or WORKING WITHOUT COFFEE IS SLEEPING) being used by a random stranger. People are not always good at sharing what belongs to them, but they are also not so great at sharing things that belong to everyone.

A friend and I recently went out for lunch at a busy café. We selected a table that had just been vacated; I plonked myself down in the seat, but my friend took a moment to move the chair and replace it with another from a table close to us—a chair that hadn't just had a person sitting in it.

"What are you doing?" I asked.

"I can't stand a warm chair," he replied. "I hate the thought of another person's ass cheeks being on a chair before mine. A cold chair is always best."

This is not unusual. I have several clients who will move the chairs in my office so they are not sitting on one that a person just left. "Another person's bum heat! It's just gross," one client told me with conviction.

This is amplified for people when using public toilets. Toilet seats (particularly in public bathrooms) are avoided by many, and some people go to extreme lengths never to sit where another person's naked bum has been. Mai, a true germophobe, refused to drink liquids during the day and would "hold it in" rather than use any toilet other than their own.

"Even at home, if someone has been to the toilet just before me, I hover," they tell me. "There's no way I am sitting on that seat."

Humans are a strange bunch. Some hate the double dip; others don't think twice about biting the corn chip and sticking it back in the hummus. Some people will jump into a hot tub without a second thought; others view it as flaked-human-skin soup. Some people can sleep in sheets and pillows that have been used by many, while others imagine a crime scene of sweat and bodily fluids.

(The manager at a hotel where I often stay told me that mattresses are changed every five to seven years, and in the time between, up to two thousand people might sleep on the same mattress. That concoction of human cells must keep the dust mites happy!)

The thought that someone has used what you are now using

might be upsetting, or it might have the opposite effect—some people form deep emotional attachments to objects specifically because they have been preowned.

I wear my grandmother's wedding ring and I love it. When I first got her ring after she died, it was so thin that it had split, as she had been wearing it every day for more than sixty years. That ring reminds me of her—her warmth and cuddles, ginger biscuits and caramels.

I bet you can think of a sentimental object that has a special meaning for you too. These kinds of objects might not be worth much money, but they are priceless in terms of the memories they hold and the stories they tell. People keep old crockery, letters and birthday cards, the ribbons they won in third grade, and the tenor saxes that they haven't played since they were twelve.

I'm attached to my gran's ring, but I have never once thought, *I wonder how Gran's ring will feel if I don't wear it?*

Objects are just objects—except when they're not. Any child will tell you that their toys are not just "things." Kids all over the world have relationships with their toys. My six-year-old neighbor's bedroom looks like the scene in *E.T.* when E.T. hides among a multitude of plush toys. My neighbor also owns piles and piles of plush toys, although they're not in piles— they are all lined up facing the middle of the room "so they can see what's going on," she told me.

"Sometimes when I go to school, I'll let some look out the window so that they can see me coming home." Each of her toys has a name and each has its own personality. She has a couple of favorites that have a special spot on her bed, "but I play with all of them," she said. "I would never want any of them to feel left out."

Children think that their toys are alive. The Toy Story movies are built on this idea. Toys have feelings and need to be cared for. Children will cry if their toys are hurt or request Band-Aids for them if they fall. Many children struggle if they have to throw out their old toys, fearing that they will feel abandoned or unloved. This is a natural part of emotional and social development. It helps children to imagine the feelings of others and learn how to respond to a wide range of emotions and situations.

My daughter had a plush tree frog that she was given when she was a newborn. She slept with this frog every day throughout her childhood and carried it with her everywhere. She would fall asleep scratching at the frog's green fur until slowly but surely the fur fell out in clumps. My father was losing his hair at the time, and my daughter called his balding head his "love patch"; she believed my mother must have scratched my father's hair out with all her love.

Most of us grow out of thinking our toys are real, but for a large number of autistic adults, toys and other inanimate objects remain "alive" and continue to have feelings. Objects may have genders and personalities and be considered friends or family. This is known as object personification, where human characteristics are given to nonhuman things.

"It can be debilitating," Sadie tells me during an appointment. "I worry all day long. I worry in the morning when I'm making a cup of tea. Which tea bag should I take out of the box? What if I pick the wrong one? What if that tea bag wants to spend more time with the others and isn't ready to be used? And don't get me started on if their strings are entwined! I would never break those tea bags apart."

She rotates through cups so that no cup feels unloved, and she restacks the plates so that no one plate is constantly on the bottom. When she is shopping, if there are only two items left on the shelf, she will buy both even if she only needs one because she doesn't want one to be left on its own.

"And I hate it when someone tells me they have lost

something!" (I bite my tongue and don't tell her that in the past month I have lost two pairs of glasses and my wallet.) "When someone loses something, I remember, and the next time I see them, I ask if it has been found, even if there have been months in between. I can't stop thinking about the thing feeling lost and afraid and never being found."

After Heidi told me how concerned she was about the feelings of hotel beds, she added, "It's exactly the same with washing machines in a shared laundry. Imagine the thousands of clothes from those thousands of people that the machine has had to cope with. Those machines must be exhausted with all the work they've had to do, and no one even cares. I would never want to add to the washing machines' pain."

Washing machines and hotel beds in Heidi's mind had been abused! And when I thought about it, it made me slightly sad too. "Maybe you could be nice to the bed, Heidi? Maybe you could show it compassion?" And although I couldn't believe these words were coming out of my mouth, I did know that for Heidi, demonstrating kindness to a bedroom ensemble was essential.

So Heidi and I devised a plan and wrote out a list of things for her to buy so she could stay at the hotel. A new mattress topper that no one had ever used (or hurt) to go on top of the hotel mattress. New sheets and pillowcases covered in bright, sunny colors. A scented candle to fill the air with the smell of calming, sleepy lavender. Heidi would treat the bed with the respect and kindness it deserved.

Heidi texted me the next day: *I stayed*, the text read.

I smiled to myself. As I put my phone down, I saw a potted plant out of the corner of my eye.

"Oh, you poor old thing," I said out loud. "You're dying of thirst."

# 5

# Elliot's Clock

Elliot and his mom entered the room in a flap. They were unhappy with each other, and this feeling radiated from both of them. Elliot, at seventeen, was dressed in a suit that did not quite fit. His jacket was hanging off his skinny shoulders and his huge hands protruded far beyond the length of the sleeves. Elliot always dressed in a suit and had a collection of secondhand pin-striped, single-breasted, and sports blazers. He was dapper, while his mom was the opposite. She was disheveled, with uncombed hair and her morning coffee staining her shirt.

Elliot and his mom had started coming to see me so that she could gain a greater understanding of his recent autism diagnosis. But more often than not, I spent their appointments trying to explain the differences between their viewpoints rather than their neurologic systems.

"We're not really speaking to each other today." Elliot's mom bristled as she took a seat. "Elliot has been yelling and swearing at me, saying that we were going to be late. But I was well aware of what time the appointment was."

Elliot's frustration could be felt across the room. "I hate

being late," he snapped at his mother. "You said one o'clock but we didn't leave at one o'clock. You were late. You're always late."

"But I told you that we'd leave *around* one," his mom responded. "I told you every single time you asked."

Every single *time*. I heard this word, and it rang like the shocking sound of my alarm at six a.m. Einstein knew that time was relative—but do the rest of us?

Time is mysterious. It is hard to comprehend the time it takes for light from the stars to reach the Earth or that the smallest measurement of time is "Planck time"—it takes trillions of Planck times to blink! How weird and wonderful is that?

We all perceive the world differently. We each have differing perceptions of color, taste, touch, and sound. How individuals perceive time differs, because time is based on how they feel about it.

There are members of my family who watch the clock and others who have no idea that the minutes are ticking by. I fall into the second group. I have to admit that I'm always late. I don't mean to be, and as I get older, I fight against it, but it's an element of my personality. I have missed buses, have had my name called over the loudspeaker at international airports, and have narrowly made it to weddings just ahead of the bridal party. I'm late for the dentist, for dinners, and for yoga classes. (Strangely, I am never late for movies, as one of my pet peeves is to miss the beginning.) This is exasperating for everyone around me. I'm sure that I'm told that meetings are scheduled for half an hour earlier than they actually are, just so I get there at the right time.

But I'm never late with intent. As Marilyn Monroe said, "I have tried to change my ways but the things that make me late are too strong and too pleasing." My strongest and most pleasing reason for lateness is people. I just love a chat, and living in a small town means running into lots of people I know while I'm on my way from one place to another.

"Only three people, Mom" is what my daughter used to say to me when we left the house together. This was her rule. A quick trip to the shops to pick up a few things would turn into a couple of hours, as I invariably needed to talk to every person I encountered. My daughter would pace and sigh and throw me glares whenever the words "Oh, hi!" came out of my mouth. People make me late for people, but I really do respect the people I am trying to get to too!

Being on time is perceived as a sign that you are aware of other people's needs, and being late is seen as a sign of disrespect. But perhaps latecomers aren't disrespectful; maybe they're just overly optimistic. The tardy can often be overconfident about how much can be jammed into a short amount of time. They believe they can shower, get dressed, pack their bags, and drive a distance of twenty-five miles all in fifteen minutes. These are the people for whom teleporting needs to be invented.

Perfectionists, strangely, can also be perpetually late. Everyone knows that person who just needs to unload the dishwasher or put clothes in the washing machine before they can get out the front door. This type of person often hates being late, but the pull to have things "just so" before leaving home works against them.

To combat this, some people try to tightly organize their time and plan their days from the moment they wake up to the moment they go to sleep. Time management is a skill, and people who possess it often have great techniques for getting to the right place at the right time. They might set their clocks to be ten minutes fast and live in "unreal time"; their diaries and calendars might be color-coded; they might set alerts and reminders on their phones; they might get up half an hour early just so they have extra time for any mishaps that might occur.

My grandfather always gave himself time, lots of it. When he traveled to visit my parents, he arrived at the train station two hours before departure. He had spent his life punching a clock, and he believed that time (and trains) stopped for no one. He preferred to sit on a bench at the station for hours before the whistle blew rather than risk missing the train. I have his watch, but, unfortunately for my timely friends, I've never worn it.

Time can cause many people anxiety. "It's better to be ten minutes early than one minute late" is how one person described the stress of lateness to me. This anxiety can wake people during the night just to check the clock or to make sure that they actually did set the alarm (but if you have time anxiety, you have *always* set the alarm).

For autistic people who love systems, routine, and certainty, time can create stress. This stress can come from the rush and apprehension of working to a set time on the clock (daily time). It can stem from the concern of what might or might not happen tomorrow (future time) or from the anxiety that there's not enough time in life, and that it is all slipping away (existential time). If this is how you think of time, of course you'll always be worried about what time it is.

While some people are always aware of the time, others have no sense of it.

Ivy was late for every appointment that she ever had with me. This wouldn't have been an issue, but as an over-crammer myself, I'd often book client appointments with barely a gap between them. Ivy's lateness triggered a ripple effect that affected every person after her, which didn't go down well, especially with those who scheduled their days to the minute.

"I don't even know that time is passing," she said. "I get completely lost in what I am doing, particularly when I'm doing the things I love." Ivy loved all types of Japanese arts and crafts. She was adept at ikebana (the art of flower arranging), produced beautiful *shodo* (ink calligraphy), and was passionate about origami.

"I'm trying to make a lion. Not the simple one—the replica of the Lion King. It has nearly eighty folds."

Ivy's brain made it difficult for her to shift gears, particularly when she was deep in the tucks and creases of origami. While her fingers were dexterous, time slipped through them.

Many neurodivergent people talk about having no perception that time is passing when they are hyper-focused. Their concentration may be so intense that day becomes night and night becomes day without their noticing. Athletes, artists, and gamers talk about being "in the zone," and psychologists call this state of being "flow." When people are fully immersed in what they are doing, everything surrounding them falls away. This is the joy of hyper-focus.

Your perception of time changes depending on how engaged you are and how old you are. Do you ever think, *Where has the year gone?* Or can you remember as a child feeling like a school semester took forever? Adults and children perceive time differently, and people also perceive time as fast or slow depending on their moods. When you are enjoying what you're doing, your brain releases chemicals that make you feel like time is passing more quickly. When the levels of these chemicals decrease, time seems to slow to a snail's pace. There are seldom happy chemicals in your brain when you're stuck in a traffic jam.

No one likes to wait. No one enjoys a long queue or waiting for a doctor to call with test results or even waiting for the toast to pop up. We hate waiting because we usually don't know when the wait will end. But one person's idea of an appropriate wait time might be completely different from another's.

Even the word *wait* made Tyler livid. He was one of my students in the high-school classroom that in those days—the early 1990s—was called the Emotionally Disturbed Unit. (How horrific is that?) The classroom was filled with young people whose names were followed by initials indicating their diagnoses: ASD, ADHD, ODD, OCD, PTSD. I loved Tyler. He was red-haired and freckled with big buck teeth. He had a wonderful sense of humor and was a born entertainer who could do impressions of all the staff; he loved to crack jokes. At that time, I was into flowing dresses and flowery pants, and not a single day went by without him saying, "Miss, you forgot to get out of your pajamas again."

Tyler was on the breakfast program. The school provided breakfast to encourage students to come to school, but Tyler didn't need encouragement. He loved school and the security of it. Tyler's home was not safe. At fifteen years old, he would couch-surf at various friends' houses when his own home was too volatile or spend weeks at a time in and out of youth shelters. He slept in cars and tents and, often, the beanbags in the corner of the classroom. I once found Tyler washing his underwear in the bathroom after school because he had not had a stable place to stay in weeks.

Tyler was a storyteller, but a lot of what he said could not be taken as fact. According to him, he had been on the biggest roller coaster in the country, parachuted out of planes, dived with sharks, run a marathon, and won a contest by eating eight meat pies in one sitting.

He once told me about a fox fur he owned. In his story, he had killed the fox with a slingshot, removed the pelt, cured it, and tanned it, and this fur was now his most prized possession. We lived in the city, and I wasn't 100 percent convinced of Tyler's hunting skills, but I listened with interest. "Wow, Tyler, I'd love to see it," I said. I thought nothing more about it until a few weeks later.

I was in the middle of a discussion with another student about why bringing ninja throwing stars to school was not a good idea when Tyler burst into the classroom with a fox fur wrapped around his shoulders.

"Miss," he called out, trying to attract my attention. "*Miss!*"

"Wait, Tyler," I responded with force in my tone.

And all hell broke loose. I've been called a few names in my life, but Tyler spat names at my face along with actual spit. He walked out, slamming the classroom door behind him, and I was left with the ninja throwing stars in my hands and the stars of hurt and confusion in my eyes.

During a calmer moment, we talked. "I'd planned to show you for weeks," he said. "I finally got to bring the fur, and you didn't even want to see it!"

"I did, Tyler. I did want to see it," I assured him.

"B-but you said *wait*," he stammered.

And then he explained his experience of "the wait." He told me that when a grown-up said, "Wait," that always meant the end of the conversation. For Tyler, when grown-ups said, "Wait," it meant that they weren't interested, and they never came back to finish the discussion. For Tyler, the word *wait* had no end; it didn't have a time limit.

"Just a minute" is never a minute. "Give me a sec" is never a second. "In a moment" is never just a moment. When you are communicating your perception of time to another person, you need to precisely communicate your idea of a minute, a second, or a moment, because the concept of time is different for all of us.

\* \* \*

"Every single time you asked, I said that we'd leave around one," Elliot's mom repeated.

I quickly grabbed a piece of paper and a pen and drew a clockface on it. "When you say 'around one,' what do you mean?" I asked Elliot's mom. "Can you draw it?"

"Oh, y'know . . . just around about then," she said. She took the pen from my hand and drew her idea of what *around one* meant.

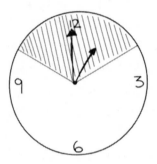

"And you, Elliot, what's 'around one' for you?" I asked, giving him the pen.

And he drew . . .

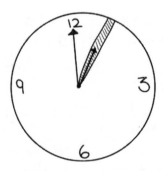

Elliot and his mom looked at each other. "Your 'around one' is not *around* one," Elliot stated.

Elliot's mom was just as surprised. "And your 'around one' has no 'around'—it *is* one!" she replied.

Einstein said time was relative, but he also said it was an illusion. Maybe we need to remember this. Some of us may be having a hard time, wasting time, or having the time of our lives. Our awareness and perceptions of the world we live in are as varied as we are.

# 6

# Dylan's Hallway

Dylan towered over the staff at school. The lanky and long-limbed sixteen-year-old's arms and legs were completely out of proportion with the rest of his body.

Dylan was a student at a high school for people with intellectual disabilities, and I was a teacher there. It was my first teaching experience in a school like this and I was learning on the job. I had a number of role models on the team of experienced, multidisciplined staff—teachers, occupational and speech therapists, and nurses, as we had many students with complex medical needs. But it was the two hundred students at that school who taught me the most. I was learning in the deep end, and what I didn't have in knowledge and experience, I made up for with enthusiasm and curiosity.

Dylan was in my homeroom. He had no speech but made a constant *clok-clok-clok* sound as he clicked his tongue against the roof of his mouth. It filled the classroom like a metronome. Just as some people hum or whistle when they're happy, this was Dylan's way of expressing happiness.

I loved that sound.

Dylan was mild-mannered and good-natured. He would approach me from behind and sniff my hair or gently play with the skin on my elbows. He loved to roll that knobbly flesh between his fingers — and, let's face it, it is quite fun, that weird bit of skin. He was a collector of pencils but he didn't write with them; Dylan would hold a pencil close to his eye (just his left eye) and roll it again and again in his peripheral vision. He particularly liked hexagon-shaped pencils that rippled as they were spun. He was a gentle giant.

There was, however, one big problem that stopped Dylan's tongue-clicking in its tracks. This problem literally floored him, as if he had been Tasered — he would drop to the ground and lay frozen with his muscles tensed. One staff member suggested that it happened for "no apparent reason," but of course, there had to be a reason. *No one* collapses without a cause, although there appeared to be no logic to it. Days and even weeks could go by without incident and then — *bam!* — Dylan was on the floor. This might happen several times a day for days in succession, or it might be sporadic, here one day and gone the next.

No one wanted to see Dylan like this, but we couldn't work out exactly what was causing "the drop." It was a mystery that we needed to solve, and it took a team of sensory detectives to do it.

Our senses are incredible. They perceive all that surrounds us and all that is within us. We use our senses every second of the day, and it's through our senses that we form a picture of the world.

Each person has a unique interpretation of sensory stimuli. Take the sound of cicadas, for example. These insects are small but they can bring some people a huge amount of joy and others great agitation. Personally, I think they're the best. Not the insects themselves—they are kind of nasty-looking—but the sound they make. Cicadas are a choir of buzzing and humming. They make different sounds to call to one another, to attract each other, and to celebrate once they have mated. Cicadas can flex and contract muscles in their abdomen so fast that, in a chorus, their vibrations sound continuous to our human ears. For me, they are the sound of summer, picnics, and sunset swims. They are the sound of happiness.

But cicadas can drive others to the brink of despair. I went away on holiday with someone who became so upset, he screamed at these unseen insects through a screen door, "*For fuck's sake, will you just shut up!* I can't hear myself think." He described the sound as screeching violins or the background noise in a grisly scene in a horror movie, a constant Norman Bates–at–the–shower–curtain. He hated cicadas and they made him incredibly irritable.

We learn from an early age about the five senses—sight, hearing, smell, touch, and taste. But we also have three internal senses: proprioceptive, vestibular, and interoceptive. The proprioceptive sense tells you where your body is in relation to space and the objects around you; it gives you an awareness of your strength and movement. The vestibular sense informs you about your balance, motion, and gravity; it alerts you when you are falling. The interoceptive sense tells you what is happening inside your body; it's that sensation that lets you know when you are hungry or full, hot or cold, or need to pee.

All of our senses receive information from specific receptors; these are the starting points of sensory processing. Inside the ear, little hairs vibrate with sound waves; in the eye, the retina senses light; and the nose has specialized receptors that pick up on all the smelly molecules from the outside world. These receptors process changes in the environment and within the body and send messages to a very clever part of the brain called the thalamus. The thalamus then sends the messages it receives from the receptors out to the other parts of the brain where the sensory information can be interpreted.

Receptors are great at sending the right amount of information based on what they are receiving. If light is bright, the visual receptors send more information than they do in the dark. If you are walking on pebbles or uneven ground, the proprioception receptors send more information than they would if you were walking on a flat floor. But some people respond so strongly to sensory information that they become hypersensitive; they may feel like the princess in "The Princess and the Pea" if even one grain of sand or one crumb is in the bed. On the flip side, some people respond only minimally to sensory information and are hyposensitive; even if the sheets are filled with sand or the remnants of a croissant, they sleep soundly. Just ask a pregnant woman about her heightened sensitivity to smell or someone with an extreme hangover about how the room spins when he raises his head—that's hypersensitivity; the senses are overreacting to information. Alternatively, ask a person who moves like a sloth in the morning about the importance of a cup of coffee and a shower to get revved up—that's hyposensitivity; the senses are underreacting.

Some neurotypical people can be hypersensitive and hyposensitive at different points in the day, but neurodivergent people can be consistently one or the other. For autistic people, one or two senses (or more) can be constantly hyperactive or hypoactive all day every day. For those who are hypersensitive, sensory processing is like putting the receptors on steroids. Tags in clothes feel like razors on the skin, and seams in socks hurt. Buttons and zippers and collars are a constant distraction, and having hair brushed or washed or cut can be agonizing. One drop of water on a shirt might require an immediate wardrobe change. But for those who are hyposensitive, gooey substances on the skin may go completely unnoticed. Food may remain around the mouth or snot left running from the nose because it is not felt there. Changes in body temperature might not be recognized, and wearing a T-shirt might seem just fine on a below-freezing day. For some, pain thresholds are so high that they might not notice they are hurt; for others, pain thresholds are so low that even a paper cut can be excruciating.

Personally, I am hypersensitive to smell. I'm set off in the perfume section of any department store. This section is often strategically placed at the store's entrance to entice shoppers with its welcoming floral and woody scents. I enter this space like a person preparing to be bombarded by rotten-egg gas. Perfume is synonymous with sensuality and pheromones and attraction; these are smells people seek. But some perfumes are just not good! Some are created from cheap chemicals that sting the eyes and give rise to headaches. When I enter the perfume section, I never stop and smell the roses.

I have worked in places where certain scented products were banned. No fragrant shampoo or deodorant or aftershave could be worn. In one school, a particularly hypersensitive boy brought about a total ban on bananas. This young man would gag and retch at the smell of an even slightly ripe banana. You know that smell—school bags might be filled with bananas that have been there for days, if not weeks, and finding these discarded mushy fruits can bring even the "iron guts" among us to our knees. This kid could sit in the front office and sniff out a banana anywhere within the school building—and project his disgust in the form of vomit across the office walls.

But some smells can create deep calm. I have worked with occupational therapists who place Popsicle sticks dipped in a range of different scents (vanilla, lavender, peppermint) into Ziploc bags for their clients. A person might use these scents to calm the senses in times of chaos. I watched one young girl sitting through a school assembly surrounded by a hundred or so other children happily reach into her "smell bag" and sniff her way through the principal's weekly update.

Then there's taste. We all know fussy eaters and it's almost a rite of passage for children to reject food. But for those who are hypersensitive to the taste or texture of food, the sensations of eating can be unbearable.

Hypersensitivity to taste runs in my family. One family member likes all foods to be separated and considers different ingredients mixed together in one dish horrendous. Any combination of sweet, salty, sour, bitter, and umami is too complex for her to decipher; there is no way that she would ever put maple syrup and bacon together. Another relative needs vegetables cut into tiny pieces; the texture of large chunks makes a dish inedible. These family members are not children; they are in their twenties, so they can prepare their own food and cook what they like as well as communicate their needs to others. For many neurodivergent people, this is more complicated.

At thirty-two years old, Rosie ate only things that were white or yellow. She was so hypersensitive that foods with more flavor beyond the extreme end of bland left her in a spin. She ate only spaghetti with cheese, chicken nuggets, and Teddy Grahams (honey-flavored). And her sense of taste was so acute that she could eat only one brand of spaghetti, one brand of cheese, one brand of nuggets, and one brand of cookies. She could tell the difference between brands even when she was blindfolded. What a person eats is completely up to them, but the body needs specific kinds of nutrition to survive. Due to Rosie's hypersensitivity, we needed to find the blandest, whitest multivitamins available. Now, this is a challenge for anyone who wants to take it on!

Senses can also collide in unique ways. I met Katie when she sought counseling for a breakdown in a relationship. During the first appointment she explained that she would become distracted by my words. When Katie heard words, she would see them as colors. This amazing crossover of senses is called synesthesia. The senses become intertwined, and one sense is experienced through another.

People with synesthesia may taste shapes or see sounds. Some see words or letters in colors; some, like Katie, hear words and see them as colors. For Katie, not every word had a color attached, but a majority of them did. The word *home* was warm dirty pink, *hurt* was burnt orange, and *celebrate* was iridescent green. I loved talking with Katie but I had to remain conscious of the words I used, as they had the potential to run into an incomprehensible, murky-colored slurry. I asked her about the colors of my favorite words: *shimmer, lullaby, tenderness,* and *rendezvous.* Katie quickly picked up that the words I was tossing around were the ones I liked the sound of.

"You don't have synesthesia, Jodi," she said. "For you, the sound of the word is just the sound."

And this is true, but I often think of Katie when I hear my parents crack the nine-letter word puzzle in the daily newspaper. I sometimes wonder what color that word would be.

The way our senses work tells us the story of where we are,

who we are, and how to look after ourselves. We all feel and interact with the world differently, and we need to remind ourselves that this fundamental component of the human brain is unique for each of us. We don't need to just walk in other people's shoes—we need to get into other people's senses.

And understanding Dylan's senses was exactly what we had to do to support him and figure out why he'd suddenly drop. When a person who is nonspeaking expresses discomfort or distress, you must jump out of your own way of sensing the world. You must experience the world through that person's unique sensory profile.

Determining what was hurting Dylan did not happen overnight. It took a great deal of trial and error and a team of people throwing around ideas.

Someone noted that Dylan always dropped in the same hall and the same spot, which was just outside a bathroom. The bathroom was huge. It contained several toilets, including wheelchair-accessible toilets, personal-care changing tables, showers, and a laundry with washing machines and dryers. It was at the door of this place of sensory overload that Dylan would fall.

Although he did not have speech, Dylan communicated with us very clearly when he flung himself to the floor. Each time, he would lie frozen with his hands clasped tightly over his ears. We knew he was protecting himself from a sound. But which one?

Maybe it was the washing machine? We turned it on and watched when Dylan passed the bathroom—nothing. We tried the dryer—nothing. Maybe it was the combination of the two? Also nothing. It took weeks. We watched Dylan and noted what was taking place inside that bathroom every time he walked in the hallway. What things were on? Which were off? It was a process of elimination. Slowly but surely, we struck sound after sound off the list.

The changing tables in the bathroom were similar to massage tables and were used for students who needed personal-care support. The tables were raised and lowered with levers. Maybe it was the sound of the tables being adjusted that Dylan couldn't cope with? If the tables were being levered from one position to another as we passed the bathroom, we kept our eye on Dylan... nothing.

Until someone turned on the fan.

Above the changing table closest to the hallway was a large exhaust fan. This fan, like all exhausts, sucked and whirred and spun. It struck us like a lightning bolt after weeks of deduction: Dylan was being knocked flat by the fan. But the fan did not affect Dylan every time it was on. He was not bothered by the fan when the changing table was at its lowest; it was only when the table was raised and the fan was on. The air pressure between table and fan changed then, and with this, the sound waves of the fan changed pitch. It was this particular sound that had Dylan falling to the floor.

This took place years before noise-canceling headphones became widely available, so we did what we needed to do—we turned the fan off.

The senses—all of them—are how we make *sense* of all that is surrounding us and within us. When some people smell something rotten, they might gag; when some hear the sound of metal on metal, they might clench their teeth; when you sink into a warm bath with muscles that are aching, you might exhale with relief. How wonderful is it that some of us love oysters and olives and some of us eat only plain pasta with cheese?

Some people can't go to sleep if they can hear a tap dripping from the other end of the house, and others think rain on the roof is a lullaby. The sound of cicadas may make some people bristle, and the perfume department can make some people swoon. All each of us needs to do, the most important thing, is be sensitive to how others experience the world.

# 7

# Sally's Food Court

Sally and I were in our early twenties when we met. I was a disability support worker and I'd been matched with her because we were of similar age. Sally wore clothes that were covered in riotous patterns, all thrown together with abandon. She loved shirts with black-and-white geometrics, skirts that rippled with flowers, leaves, and birds, brightly colored socks, and glittery shoes. We were different in our dress sense but we had many other things in common. We both loved to read, but while I loved all types of books, Sally read only the Earth's Children series, to the point that when she talked about Ayla (a character who was raised by Neanderthals), I thought at first she was Sally's friend. We both loved to walk and walk far. We both loved movies and wholeheartedly agreed that eating ice cream (choc-tops) at the cinema was a must. And we both loved sushi. We *loved* it. We could eat sushi for every meal, including breakfast.

Once a week, Sally and I met up and headed out for the day. Our routine was the same every time. We would toss a coin to decide whether we would take a walk or see a movie, but we'd always start with sushi.

Sally insisted that we eat at the same cheap and cheerful sushi shop at the local mall, and she always ate the exact same combination: a California roll and a teriyaki chicken roll with soy sauce and ginger (but never wasabi). We loved our routine, but one day something went terribly wrong.

Sally's face was contorted; tears rolled down her cheeks. She looked like someone in the midst of a major battle. We were in the food court at the mall, and Sally was in agony. This didn't make sense. We had been here every week for months, and Sally had never looked like she was in a war zone before.

Sally began banging her head on the table—not hard, not violently, but rhythmically, the way a person might knock water out of their ears after swimming. I watched as her body moved into a state of terror. Her eyes were squeezed shut; her arms covered her head as if she were trying to protect herself from incoming shrapnel; her legs were shaking; and she was hyperventilating. I could literally see her heart pounding.

"Sal, tell me what's happening," I pleaded. "How can I help?"

But Sally couldn't answer me. All her energy was spent on fighting whatever melee was going on inside her head. She was falling to pieces in front of me in the food court, and I had no idea why.

We're all aware of how we pay attention to some information but ignore the rest. As I write this, the dishwasher is churning and the radio is on; the program host is chatting about the best vegetables to plant in spring. There are cars passing on the road outside, children playing a game in the yard out front, and someone is using a high-pressure hose on the driveway out back. But while I'm typing, I give all these sounds that surround me little or no regard. This is called selective attention, and most of us do it all the time.

We're bombarded with a lot of sensory information every minute of the day, and our brains latch onto what's important and overlook what's not. The thalamus has two jobs: to interpret sensory stimuli and filter this information, determining which messages from the sensory receptors are worth listening to and which can be ignored. The thalamus protects us from the onslaught of too much sensory input.

For many autistic people, the thalamus works differently, and filtering information can be difficult. Some autistic people might try hard to listen to you, but any background noise, like a child crying or a dog barking, will be given the same amount of attention as your voice, and that person's brain will try to focus on all things at once. Some people are unable to buffer the torrent of sensory information in certain environments, and when the brain does not filter the information, it becomes overloaded. The senses flooding the brain cannot be contained, and it can be overwhelming.

I live in a subtropical climate, and the heat and the sun and the wet is a smorgasbord for the senses. The days can be so humid, you feel the sweat trickling down your back and you wish for a storm, just for the relief of rain and a break from the heat. But when the rain does come, it can pelt down relentlessly for days. It rains a lot, and it rains *hard*. No laundry can be done, and the laundromats celebrate as their dryers cycle 24/7. Houses fill with mold and mildew, but windows cannot be opened to air homes out. Roads flood, and people are evacuated to higher ground, and we all impatiently wait for the sun.

It can also be dazzlingly bright here, with wide-open blue skies. The sun beats down with the type of sunshine that makes you glow and need to swim and *want* to eat salad. Those days are filled with the scent of frangipanis and the sounds of lawn mowers and laughter.

Driving on these days, you wind the window down and wish you could stick your whole head out, like a dog, and feel the breeze. You drive one-handed, with your hand resting lightly on the wheel like it's an old friend. The radio is on and your favorite songs are playing. You sing as loudly and as badly as you want in these moments, because singing loudly and badly in the car is essential in life. If you're not alone, you can listen to your friend telling you a story in the passenger seat beside you and to the classic 1980s hit on the radio and be at ease with both. You can also hear the banter of children in the back seat, and together, all three—David Bowie, your friend's conversation, and the children's chatter—are in perfect unity.

Your posture is comfortable and relaxed in the seat, and your eyes take in what is ahead as well as what is behind in the rearview mirror; in your peripheral vision, you're aware of the passing countryside. Everything is in harmony, and you're doing a dozen things at once without even realizing it.

Now imagine that a raindrop hits the windshield. Your sight sends the information to your brain. *It's beginning to rain,* the brain says. It alerts the senses: *Hey, you lot, attention is now needed.*

More raindrops fall, and the breeze becomes stronger. You turn the windshield wipers on low so you can see better, and you close the window. The rain falls harder and faster and your brain continues to turn down and tune out the senses that aren't needed so it can concentrate. Although your friend continues to talk and the children continue chatting in the back seat, you no longer listen.

When it's bucketing down, it's all systems go. The radio is now loud and annoying, so you turn it off. You adjust your hands to ten and two on the wheel and grip it with white knuckles. You don't let your eyes stray from the road.

You concentrate on only the senses that are necessary in that moment so you can focus on staying safe. As the rain beats down and the windshield wipers move through their paces to their top speed, you become hypervigilant. Your proprioceptive sense is alert; you shift in your seat; you are upright and wary. You focus solely on the road. Everything else must fall away.

The thalamus is like a mixing board for a band. Depending on the song, different instruments will be amplified or softened, and the thalamus works in much the same way. It modulates the sensory information and raises or lowers the level of sensory input so that the senses can harmonize together when the environment is safe and calm; when it is not, it might bring one or two to the foreground while letting others fade.

When things are not right, your unneeded senses start to shut down one by one, and the mixing board orients the senses to what is most important and immediate. Your nervous system tells you to be alert. Your brain tells you to pull back on the olfactory, tone down the tactile...bring it all back to acoustic. Simplify.

While the majority of neurotypical people have the ability to block out sensory information and give selective attention to only what is needed, many autistic people cannot filter their senses as quickly or easily. Autistic people can have difficulty with sensory processing because their nervous systems just take all of it in. Add a stressful situation or an environment that is overstimulating, and just when less stimulation is needed, not more, the sensory-processing systems of many autistic people become overwhelmed.

The brain perceives all of this immense input as pain. Sensory overload is torture. Just imagine not being able to escape an environment where rock music is blaring from different speakers at the same time, red lights are flashing constantly, and the air-conditioning is turned to its maximum temperature. Imagine driving in torrential rain, except your windshield wipers aren't working and you can't wind the window up and you can't turn the blaring music down. The brain cannot cope with these kinds of extremes and will send a cascade of feeling through your body. You will panic.

Back in the fluorescently lit mall, Sally was in the midst of a sensory storm, and the food court had become a hurricane.

At first, I couldn't work out what had gone wrong. We normally started our routine each week at Sally's favorite shop, and at ten a.m., there were rarely many people in the mall—but that day had been different. Sally had had a dental appointment in the morning, so our day had been pushed back a few hours. By the time we arrived at the mall, it was lunchtime, and the food court was in overdrive. While Sally tried to block out the world, I tried to unblock my neurotypical sensory filtering of the food court. I tried to see what Sally saw and hear what Sally heard.

If you visit a food court at lunchtime, let your senses take it all in. Noise comes from every direction. There are people talking *everywhere*, all in different volumes and accents and speeds. They're talking on phones. They're ordering food. Chairs are scraping, cutlery is clanging, and trays are being bashed. There is munching and crunching and slurping through straws. There is music and advertising blasting through loudspeakers. And then there's the many smells of all the various foods—the burgers and burritos and french fries and doughnuts—as well as the smells of all the perfumes and deodorants and bodies. There's movement and color and lights, all twisting and blinking and blurring.

Sally's capacity to filter her senses disintegrated, and her brain was under siege. Her senses were sending a danger signal to her brain, and that message had gone beyond a warning. Fear had taken over her body. Sally was having a panic attack. She couldn't breathe; she had chest pain; she was trembling and sweating and dizzy.

For nearly ten minutes I watched Sally battle her sensory overload. She was being attacked from all sides, and all those years ago, I didn't understand the extent of the barrage. But I do now. I know that sensory overload is torturous, that having all your senses bombarded is harrowing.

Once Sally was calmer and able to move, I took her hand and guided her through the chaos of the food court, past the shops, and into the sunshine outside. There, we sat together on a bench in the open air. We sat in the world that gave us fluffy, slow-moving clouds, the swishing of leaves in trees, and a gentle breeze. Sally's body relaxed and she closed her eyes.

"Just breathe deep, Sal" was all I had to offer. "Just breathe."

Modifying an environment to make it accessible for neurodivergent people is not always easy, but it is possible. If you can consider the world from others' point of view—when you stand still just for a moment and perceive any space, any place, through the senses of another—what can you see? What can you smell? What can you touch? What can you hear? That day,

Sally taught me that sushi in a food court at lunchtime is, just like driving in the pouring rain, best avoided!

We can't always know what impact an unknown environment will have on someone. Sometimes you get stuck in the eye of the sensory storm, and all you can do is wait for the storm to pass. The best we can do in moments like these is help one another find a way back to the calm.

# 8

# Melanie's Hair

M elanie had golden-brown wavy hair that fell to her waist. It was a defining feature: "Oh, you know Melanie—the one with the fabulous hair." That isn't to say that she didn't have other features that could have been used as descriptors: "Melanie, the one with the blue glasses that match her eyes." "Melanie, the one who wears the Indian bracelets that jingle as she walks." "Melanie, the one who always—and I mean *always*—wears black tights and a green top. You know, *that* Melanie."

But it was the hair that people remembered, partly because it was so beautiful and partly because Melanie spent so much time playing with it.

Melanie came to see me because she was having difficulty with her body image, and this was affecting her relationships and sexual intimacy. Talking to someone about sexuality can fill most of us with trepidation, and Melanie was no exception. Her nervous mannerisms were noticeable moments after she arrived at my office. She sat in the middle of the three-seater couch and began to twirl her hair. With her right hand, she gathered a lock of hair up close to the root and twisted it around her finger, a graceful movement that traveled all the way down the length of her hair. When she let it go, it formed a perfect ringlet. And then she did it again. And again. And again. The same piece of hair. Melanie did not stop twirling her hair for even one moment that we were together.

"Hey, Melanie," I said after she had been to see me a few times, "when you're playing with your hair, do you know you're doing it?"

"Oh, is it bad?" she asked. "Am I not supposed to do it?"

I think my jaw dropped. Who on earth would tell another person that they were not allowed to play with their own hair? "It's your hair—you can do whatever you like with it," I assured her. "I just wondered how it makes you feel when you do it."

I love the expression "jumping for joy." Our bodies reflect how we feel. Have you ever watched people when they're excited? They jump up and down and wave their arms around. It's a natural reaction to the world being wonderful. And have you ever watched a child cutting with scissors? While concentrating on a new (and potentially dangerous) task, many kids will stick out their tongues and move them the same way they move the scissors. Or have you ever sat with people who constantly crack their knuckles, chew the ends of their pencils, or bite their nails?

Repetitive movement is something that we all do. People twiddle their thumbs, snap their fingers, or rub their beards. We make these movements when we are bored or lost in thought but also when we're anxious or uncomfortable. They're often subtle and done unconsciously, but these movements can be more readily seen and have been pathologized in autistic people because of their frequency.

Sometimes called *stimming*—short for *self-stimulatory behavior*—repetitive movements include hand-flapping, finger-flicking, repeated blinking, teeth-grinding, palm-rubbing, hair-twirling, or rocking back and forth. Historically, it was believed that stimming hindered people's learning and that autistic people stimmed to avoid situations. Stimming was considered "not okay" and something that needed to be stopped. But when did people start thinking of rocking as bad?

Without thinking about it, whenever I pick up a baby, I rock and sway my body from side to side, and my hips move from left to right and back again. All of us know instinctively that rocking soothes, otherwise we wouldn't spend so much money on swaying cribs, baby bouncers, and baby swings. We buy rocking chairs for the gentle lulling of a newborn baby but also to provide comfort for aging grandparents. People rock themselves when they're upset or distraught. We rock our whole lives because it calms the central nervous system.

The central nervous system—the brain and the spinal cord—takes in sensory information and sends orders out to the body. At the base of the brain is the brain stem, which connects to the spinal cord. The spinal cord carries the messages back and forth between the brain and all of the nerves in the body. This incredible system of nerves helps the parts of the body communicate with one another and reacts to changes outside and inside the body. But for autistic people, the messages can sometimes be sent too quickly or too slowly.

Stimming has many benefits, including regulating the central nervous system. It can help people manage overwhelming sensory information. For people who are hypersensitive, stimming can reduce sensory overload, as it focuses the brain on just one constant, reassuring, and comforting movement. For people who are hyposensitive, stimming can wake up the senses by providing more feedback. Stimming can enliven the senses. It can also help people center themselves when they're anxious or demonstrate elation or glee.

Not all stims are physical, though—most of us have verbal habits too. When I first went to university to become a teacher, a lecturer filmed each of us running a class for our fellow students. The lecturer encouraged us to watch ourselves and pay attention not to the content of what we said but to our mannerisms. I started nearly every sentence with *um*. It was excruciating to hear. I imagined the kids I'd be teaching in a high-school classroom taking bets on how many times I'd say it.

All of us use verbal or vocal fillers to give ourselves time to gather our thoughts. We say *right* or *you know*, and it's hardly noticeable unless it becomes exaggerated in its repetition. I have one friend who sighs when there's a break in the conversation and another who adds *okay* to the beginning and end of nearly every sentence. And nearly every teenager overuses *like*: "Or, like, when I, like, saw her in the street after school, she, like, asked me to go to her house."

Some neurodivergent people repeat words and phrases not just as fillers but because the words sound good or feel good in the mouth. I knew one young boy who said the word *marshmallow* over and over when he was happy and another who said, "I'm completely taken aback" whenever he started a new activity. Groaning, squealing, clearing the throat, and smacking the lips are all vocal stims.

We use repetitive mannerisms throughout the day but more often when we're uneasy or nervous. I once took an autistic student from the school where I was working to a youth mental-health conference for some "real-world" learning. The university lecture hall was filled with more than four hundred people, all packed in like sardines. The only two seats available were in the middle of a row. We shuffled our way along an aisle as people shifted their legs sideways, moved their bags, and folded up the small desks attached to university chairs. This fourteen-year-old did not like crowds, and when she was anxious, she wriggled. After she sat down, she immediately started fidgeting: rummaging through the conference satchel, opening and closing the lid of her water bottle, and drumming her fingers on the armrest between us. When the first speaker started, she stopped fidgeting but her leg started to shake. Her leg was moving with so much force that it rippled the chairs around us.

"Will you *stop* moving," hissed the woman sitting next to her. (This was in the middle of a conference on adolescent mental health—ironic, really.)

I ripped a piece of paper from my notebook, took a pen from my pencil case, and passed them to my companion. She started to draw, and her body stilled immediately. I am a pen clicker, but I know pen spinners, label pickers, and paper-clip unfolders. Many of us need to play with objects to calm our nerves and help us concentrate.

We might also engage in repetitive mannerisms out of pleasure. Can you remember spinning to make yourself dizzy as a kid? Zoe was a spinner. I often thought she should have been recruited into the national ballet company. In her late teens, she was tall and strong yet light on her feet. Her calf muscles were rock solid. Zoe particularly liked to spin outside, barefoot on soft grass. She would rise onto her tippy-toes, and with her head thrown back and her arms spread like an eagle's wings, she would spin and spin and spin. After fifteen or twenty spins, Zoe would stop and then, without a single stumble, take a few steps and start again. She was on cloud nine.

While Zoe should have been in a ballet company, Grayson should have been the plate spinner in the circus. He had hundreds of spinning tops, but that wasn't all he liked to spin. As a small child he would spin the wheels on all his toys; he would spin the knives and forks on the table, and he'd turn his bowls on the side and spin them too. He loved to watch ceiling fans and standing fans, front-loader washing machines and dryers. Grayson was in seventh heaven in any laundromat. He even had his eighth birthday party at one!

Stimming for pleasure does not require any type of therapy or intervention, but there are some repetitive stims that cause physical harm. Sometimes autistic people hurt themselves in an attempt to drown out everything else. They might butt their heads against things, bite themselves, pick at their skin to the point of injury, cut themselves, or pull out their hair. Most of us will never feel a level of sensory or emotional overload so severe that the only way to block it out is by injuring ourselves. But it does happen to some people, and when it does, they need our love and support, not our judgment.

Think of a band's drummer. Everyone sees the drummer as the wild one, but it's the drummer who keeps the beat. When an autistic person is stimming, just think of the drummer. If they don't keep the beat with their stimming, their neurological pathways, just like the rest of the band, won't be able to stay in rhythm.

We all have a drummer within us, and we all have repetitive stims, but some of us are more Iron Maiden than the Beatles.

Melanie sat in silence and continued to twist her long lock of hair. I waited for her to give me a deeper understanding of how this graceful movement made her feel.

Melanie took time to process questions, and I loved to watch her do it. When asked a big question, Melanie would close her eyes and open them only when she had come to a con-clusion. She always answered with profound insight.

"When I play with my hair, I think it's like you and the way you rub your chest," she said. "Sometimes when you're listen-ing or saying something that has emotion in it, you pick up your right hand and rub the middle of your chest, like you are trying to be nice to your heart."

And as she talked, I realized the palm of my hand was smack-bang against my chest and gently circling the top of my sternum.

We all use repetitive movements to soothe ourselves when anxious, when we are deep in concentration, or just because it feels good. Are you clicking that pen, pulling that random long hair that grows on your arm, checking for split ends in your hair, or jiggling your leg right now? Sometimes you don't even know you are doing it until someone else points it out.

Maybe we need to view stimming for what it is: settling, calming, and pleasurable. And what's so wrong with that?

# 9

# Beth's Stake

*I*'m going to cut off your heads and stick them on a stake!" Beth screamed. *"I'm going to pierce your hearts with a sword and rip out your tongues!"*

Beth was like a Viking warrior without the leather, metal, and rippling muscles. Buxom and soft around the edges, she hated bras and never wore one. For Beth, comfort was key, and wires, straps, hooks, and fasteners did not align with this ideal. She wore orthopedic shoes and tracksuit pants with elastic waists and old, threadbare T-shirts. Beth was a walking catalog for comfort, but the place that she felt the most uncomfortable wasn't in a bra or a pair of heels — it was around other people.

In her early twenties, Beth had transitioned out of school and into adult services, and she was finding groups and community-based activities a challenge.

"I'm going to saw off your legs!" she had ranted during a recent group activity. "And then I'm going to gouge out your eyes!"

Beth was suspended from that group until she received therapy to get her "anger issues" under control.

"Do you think she was serious?" asked the disability-services coordinator when she called me. "Do you really think that she'd do that? She *sounded* serious…"

When we're upset or angry, we might say things we don't mean, words we wish we could take back. Sometimes what comes out of people's mouths is terrible and hurtful and not even true. In the moment, they feel justified, but once they calm down, they regret these words and seek forgiveness for the outburst. In the heat of the moment, people say things that they would never contemplate saying when they are calm.

"I hate you!" screamed my seven-year-old daughter from the top of the slide in response to being told it was time to pack up and leave the park. Hearing these three words from my child cut me to the core, but although I was hurt, I didn't react. "I hate you" is a typical part of child development and extends to the teenager slamming the bedroom door at news of an unwanted curfew. These children don't really hate their parents; they're just reacting to a situation by impulsively using the strongest, most forceful words that they can. It's the most powerful way they have to express their anger.

Unlike children and mood-swinging adolescents, adults are expected to control their emotions, particularly big ones like anger. But emotions can be like caged tigers, and when the opportunity arises, they pounce, sometimes at ridiculous times.

Just this week while I was driving, the car in front of me started fluctuating in speed and then tailgating the little car ahead of it. I saw the tailgating driver throw up his arms in exasperation, and then, with a vicious swerve, he went around the tiny yellow vehicle with the STUDENT DRIVER sign, flipped the person behind the wheel the bird, and yelled something out his window.

I once eavesdropped on a woman's phone conversation on a

bus. (This wasn't difficult, as it was quiet and filled only with the woman's voice.) She screamed at the customer-service operator, who, according to her, was solely responsible for the overcharges on her bill. And it wasn't just the bill—the call-center employee was also to blame for the passwords the woman couldn't remember.

Another time, I watched a customer in a busy café berate a waiter over the insufficient amount of bacon accompanying his eggs. "That's how much bacon comes with the big breakfast," the teenage waiter calmly stated. "You can order extra if you like." And the man lost it. "I could buy a whole pig for that price!" he sneered. The waiter was not the person who made decisions about bacon serving sizes, but he was now the person who had to stand steady and listen to Bacon Guy's long and agitated lecture on the correct amount of meat to put on a plate. In Australia, we call these episodes of adults losing their temper and acting like children "spitting the dummy." (*Dummy* is Australian for *pacifier*.)

Everyone flies off the handle on occasion. I'm a pacifist by nature; I'm not prone to big mood swings and I'm fairly even-keeled. But like most people, there are times when I lose the plot. I once threw a grapefruit at my partner's head. I was aiming straight at him, and in the moment when I threw it, I really did want to knock some sense into him. It's lucky that I have very bad aim, and he caught it, but I was horrified that I'd done it. Horrified! I'd snapped.

Emotional regulation is the opposite of catapulting citrus. Also called self-regulation, emotional regulation is the ability to think before you act. Anger can sizzle and bubble, and anger can erupt. A blast can destroy everything in its path, or, like volcanic ash, take weeks to settle.

Anger can be a shock wave of negative emotion, a torrent of

feelings, but most people have the neurological capacity to change the course of these rapids and slow the surge. They can take a moment to consider their actions and not react in a manner that is harmful to others or self-destructive. With good self-regulation, people learn to pause.

Some people are born with more even temperaments than others, but we all learn how to self-regulate. We don't expect young children to be in control of their distress; we understand that their brains are still growing and that having tantrums is part of being a child. As children grow, they are taught to deal with the stressors of everyday life and to "take a deep breath" so they can communicate their needs in a calm manner or problem-solve a difficult situation. Gaining these skills is a slow process, as the area of the brain involved in self-control is not fully developed until the teen years; some scientists believe that it's not fully developed until people are in their mid-twenties. The good news is that we can continue to change our brains throughout our lives.

Most of us are taught to stop and consider. We're taught to look before we leap and told that if we have nothing nice to say, we should say nothing at all. We're taught to ignore annoying people and walk away. We're taught to be good sports and to put ourselves in our own time-outs. We're taught to communicate our anger in an assertive but not aggressive way, and we're told to get enough food, exercise, and rest so that we are at our best. We need to continue to remind ourselves of these skills across our lifetime.

All people occasionally have trouble managing their emotions, but some neurodivergent people may struggle to monitor the feelings in their bodies and modulate their emotions due to their neurological system. Having an understanding of yourself is vital for regulating your emotions. Most of us are snappish when we are sleep-deprived or have low blood sugar.

Hunger nearly led a friend of mine to divorce over curtains. One morning before she left for work, she asked her partner to open the curtains and let some light into the house. When she returned home in the early afternoon, the curtains were still closed, and she was irate. Her partner was still in bed, and she entered the bedroom and went off.

"I asked you to do one thing! Just one! And you can't even do that! You're so lazy! You *never* do a thing to help! I have to do *everything!*" And she stormed out of the house, keys in hand, vowing never to return again.

And then she calmed down.

"Oh, it was so silly," she told me later. "I'd had such a busy morning that I hadn't eaten breakfast. I was hangry. When I got home, all I wanted to do was have some lunch." The worst of it was that her partner had had a migraine and couldn't even get out of bed. She recognized that she'd seen the world only through her "I wanted the curtains open" lens.

When we overreact, it's often because of the lens through which we view the moment. We may see the world only in black and white, and it becomes all or nothing. We make statements that start with "You always" or "You never." When we're blinded by our emotions, we cannot see the in between. Sometimes a switch has been flipped and the overreaction is based on the past, not the present. Bottled-up feelings of resentment, bitterness, and hurt can boil to the surface. All of us can be pressure cookers of emotions.

Being grumpy and flying off the handle on occasion is natural, but being constantly and consistently irritated and reactive is not. Emotional dysregulation is ongoing reactivity that is disproportional to the situation. For some people, like those living with anxiety and depression, emotional dysregulation can be part of their day-to-day struggles. It can have a major impact on a person's quality of life and relationships. If people fire up and explode regularly, they leave those around them in the wake of these emotions and often feel remorse, guilt, and regret for their outbursts.

The human brain evolved to react quickly. Nestled in the middle of it is an ancient structure: the amygdala. When the brain senses any threat, the amygdala reacts instantaneously, directing the body to fight, flee, or freeze. Thousands of years ago, this fight-flight-or-freeze response was vital, as it was all about survival. The amygdala still works to protect us from threat, and, when we're threatened, the fight response can be felt and demonstrated in a rapid outburst of anger.

The amygdala is also responsible for processing emotions, but not everyone's neural network processes emotions in the same way. For some autistic people, the split-second firing of impulses from the amygdala sends them into survival mode and doesn't give the frontal lobe, where consequences are considered, the chance to get in on the decision. Everyone knows what it feels like to have a rush of anger. In that moment you may want to shout, break something, punch something, or call someone a terrible, horrible name. But your frontal lobe should say, *Hang on a minute! Is this really a good idea?* The frontal lobe works to put the brakes on anger . . . but sometimes the brakes fail.

For some neurodivergent people, when they get angry, it's like there's a big brick wall cutting off the neurological pathway from the amygdala to the frontal lobe. A neurodivergent person's brain wiring can make them hotheaded, with limited capacity to engage the *Should I do this?* part of the brain. And if you don't have time to stop and think, you just do.

Levi was one of these people. I have worked with many clients across my thirty-year career, and I'm well aware that some people cannot control their words or actions when emotions are running high. I can visualize the wall coming up in their neurological pathways the moment it happens. Levi's wall was double-bricked and iron-enforced.

Levi was a big man; I only just reached the height of his chest. He was broad and strong and moved through his world like John McEnroe on the tennis court after a referee's decision didn't go his way. Levi came to one of our appointments after having had a very bad morning, and I made his day even worse. Levi consistently blamed those around him for the obstacles he encountered in life. "It's not my fault" was his default response for every stumbling block. He'd provide details of who or what had been the cause of the problem, but it was never, ever Levi.

That morning Levi had gotten a speeding ticket. This had nothing at all to do with *his* driving and everything to do with the "number of speeding tickets the police have to give out to reach their quota." According to Levi, the police had targeted him for their own purposes. I made the mistake of asking about personal accountability. I might have said something as dumb as "But who was driving the car, Levi?" It was like waving a red flag in front of a bull, and Levi reacted with gusto. He bulldozed the table in front of us so that papers and pens went flying, swept the books from the bookshelf, and upended a chair. This was accompanied by "Whose side are you on?" and "Are you a fucking cop?" plus a few other rage-filled words that left my back pressed against my chair. I wasn't frightened. I was watching the tennis player throw his racket in frustration, and I waited in silence. After some frantic pacing, Levi picked up his chair and sat down, still fuming but no longer foaming at the mouth. He had released his angry energy, and once it was out, the emotion dissipated. An initial display of emotional dysregulation does diminish. I just had to control *my* emotions and wait it out.

We've all heard that we should count to ten before we react when we are angry or upset, and there is science to back this up. It actually takes the chemicals and hormones released from the amygdala six seconds to dissipate. You don't need to literally count to ten; you just need to know that by pausing, you're giving the brain's frontal lobe a chance to weigh in. When a person is overreacting, it is important to remember this and stay unruffled so that you don't throw fuel on the fire. It can be very hard in the heat of the moment not to overreact, but two emotionally dysregulated, angry people are a head-on collision. It will end in tears. When a person is dysregulated, that is something they need to work on, but *your* reaction is in your control.

The spiteful words from a person's mouth, the verbal bash or the silent treatment, the slamming of doors, the breaking or smashing of objects, and the throwing of grapefruits are all signs of emotional dysregulation. I'm sure that you can name a time or two when you overreacted to a situation.

There's always a reason for a person's anger. Sometimes it comes from a place of hurt and pain. Sometimes it's a passionate objection to injustice or a response to frustration. Sometimes a person's brain is wired in such a way that it processes common, day-to-day experiences—for instance, being in a group of people—as threats. We all experience anger, and anger itself does have benefits. We *should* experience anger when threatened or insulted. We *should* experience anger when faced with injustice or exploitation. The feelings of anger can motivate us and provide us with the energy to stand up and take action against that which is not right.

Anger itself is neither good nor bad. It's how we respond to these feelings that counts. We can't live our lives being perpetually cool, calm, and collected, but we can learn to control our emotions and not have our emotions control us.

* * *

Five years after Beth threatened to put people's heads on stakes, she was working in the kitchen of an elder-care facility, and she loved to hear the stories that came with the wisdom of age. She lived with her scruffy and loyal dog and her equally scruffy and loyal boyfriend.

For Beth, learning to regulate her emotions—especially the big, difficult ones—had taken a lot of practice. She'd learned to be aware of her own reactions and why she was having them. She began to recognize and name the situations where she was most likely to lose control, such as being in a group where she hated the activity. We drew pictures of the brain and how it sends messages so she could visually understand how thoughts, feelings, and actions were connected. She practiced recognizing the first feelings of anger and breathing through them. Beth also created her own system of understanding. She visualized her anger as the fast-flowing traffic on a multilane freeway and imagined it being slowed by yield and stop signs. She would slow the feelings so that she could find the rest stop on the highway and have time to think.

By using these methods, Beth developed the tools to regulate her emotions. She even joined a Viking reenactment club full of people! Every weekend, she would charge at others waving a sword or an ax and screaming a war cry: "*Kill them all! Kill them all!*" And when the battle was over, she would sit down with the warring Vikings for a cup of tea.

"I'm a Karl," Beth told me.

"What's a Karl?" I asked.

"They're the middle-class Vikings—the farmers, the craftspeople, the warriors."

Beth is a Viking warrior after all.

# 10

# Margot's Gut

I don't understand what joy is," Margot said to me. "How do you know what it feels like?"

How do you explain the emotion of joy? As "elation, satisfaction, contentedness"? But these are all emotions too! You can't explain an emotion with more emotions...can you?

I love the curveball questions that are thrown at me by many neurodivergent people. I love the ones that make me stop and think, and sometimes I need time to really get my head around my response. "What does joy feel like?" was one of those questions.

Margot was beautiful inside and out. She could have won a facial-symmetry contest, with her big doe eyes and luscious lips, and she spoke with a lilting voice. Counseling sessions with Margot took place via video calls, and when I saw her on my computer screen, she was usually sitting holding a sheepskin rug or a plush toy, with her cat wandering in and out of view. She lived in a studio apartment in a big city and had built a community of people around her through her love of art and painting. She could have been in a Renoir.

Margot was a talker, and I felt I could listen to her for days. She was in her mid-forties and, like many autistic women, she had gotten her diagnosis later in life. Prior to being diagnosed with autism, Margot had had multiple misdiagnoses, and she was shedding some of the past words that had been attached to her. She was still finding her identity and learning what being an autistic woman meant for her.

Margot had been referred to me for support around relationships. She had been hurt many times in her life. She attracted men, but most of her relationships had not been successful. These relationships had ranged from an unloving, unhappy marriage to multiple short-term experiences. Some had ended in ghosting, and some were abusive. Despite this, Margot still believed in love. She believed that there was someone for everyone. Her description of her "someone" covered the front and back of a piece of paper in writing so tiny, it looked like the print in an old telephone book.

Margot's desired qualities in a potential partner included being loyal and dependable as well as tall and hairy. It included sharing her appreciation of nature and science, and a list of what he would bring to the relationship (financial security) and what he wouldn't (children). I loved her list (although I wasn't sure if there was a man alive who could match every one of the 146 bullet points), but I noticed there were no words relating to *her* anywhere.

"How should a relationship make *you* feel, Margot?" I asked. "Secure, comfortable, fulfilled?" Margot tilted her head, and I could see that I might as well have asked her to solve a quadratic equation.

In one appointment, Margot described a recent date with someone she had met online. "We went to a lovely restaurant," she said, "and he was easy to talk to. But the whole time, it was like I was a passenger in a car with a terrible driver, when you keep thinking that you might crash."

"Wow," I said. "You're very intuitive."

She looked at me blankly.

"That gut feeling?" I tried to explain. "That feeling in your gut that tells you something isn't quite right? That's your intuition."

"Explain to me what a gut feeling feels like," Margot said.

Another whammy!

*The weight of the world, on top of the world, cold feet, on the edge of your seat*—we have many expressions for the feelings in our bodies, but how do we learn about these emotions? Most of us know what it is to feel happy, sad, and angry, but these are only a few in the vast range of emotions that humans feel and can name.

We feel awe and excitement and pleasure. We feel despair and gloom and guilt, and we get stressed and worried and anxious. How can we distinguish among all of these? How do we know what exhilaration feels like? How do I know that my feeling of bitterness is the same as someone else's? How do we know what hope feels like?

I watched a father teaching his son to ride a bike in the park the other day. The boy was young, maybe four, and he hadn't yet mastered the art of the push and rotation of the pedals. He was determined to give it a good go, but by the time I got close to the two of them, the boy was on the ground next to the bike, trying to move the pedals with his hands. He was crying and yelling at the bike.

"This bike is stupid," he wailed. "It's broken. It doesn't work."

His father watched and for a few moments did not intervene. "Raj," he finally said. "Raj, you're frustrated."

He could have said *Raj, you're angry,* or *Raj, you're mad,* but he didn't. He named the emotion for exactly what it was. Hopefully Raj's brain would register the body feelings of frustration and link these feelings with the word. Maybe next time Raj felt a growl rise in his throat, he would be able to articulate it: "I'm frustrated."

Some children are lucky enough to have caregivers who help them develop a personal emotional dictionary. We all hear parents of young children expressing to their kids what they believe the children are feeling: "Lisa is sad"; "Ally is excited." This allows the children to imprint the feeling of these emotions into their brains so they can recall, express, and communicate these when needed.

Many people have trouble expressing their emotions or have poor emotional vocabularies. There are hundreds of words for emotions that I don't often use in everyday conversation, like *pensive, melancholy,* and *triumphant,* but I still know them. As I looked through a big list of emotions, I went back time and time again to these questions: What does dread or delight actually feel like? How would I describe it? How do I know the difference between all of these emotions?

One of my all-time-favorite emotions is anticipation—not anticipating the worst, but that feeling when you know something great is going to happen. I particularly like it when it is linked to people I love. Most people know that feeling of anticipation—when someone you have a crush on, a friend you haven't seen for a while, or a beloved family member is coming to visit. That feeling of waiting for them to arrive is the best. I love the feeling of anticipation in my body, the jittery flutter in my stomach. I'm more alert and can't sit still. My mind is filled with all that is to come, the feelings and thoughts about how I'll see them soon and be able to hug them and talk with them and sit up late into the night sharing stories. Anticipation is also why I love airports and train stations, front doors and gates. It's why I love meeting places. But I rarely stop to think about how my body *feels* anticipation, how it sends the message to my brain and my brain says, *Yep, you're anticipating, and you love this!*

Bodies do amazing things in reaction to the environment and different situations. Your central nervous system will send a shiver down your spine, increase your heart rate, or give you goose bumps. It can make your stomach churn or your eyes squeeze shut in pain. It can put a spring in your step or make you want to curl up into a fetal position. All of these body feelings and their different combinations and intensities are given names, like *scared, anxious,* and *disgusted.* But we sometimes struggle to decode these mingled sensations and name them for exactly what they are.

When I was in a waiting room this week, a young girl sat close to me watching a video on her tablet of the children's song "If You're Happy and You Know It." But this was a new version that covered many emotions. The little girl acted out all of the body movements mentioned in the song: "If you're happy and you know it, clap your hands. If you're scared and you know it, hide your eyes. If you're angry and you know it, stamp your feet." As I watched her, I realized that many of us have learned about our emotions upside down.

In school, we're taught what emotions look like—in others. We're shown pictures of other people's faces—happy faces, surprised faces, and sad faces—and asked, "What does this person feel?" But shouldn't we be taught to observe first what our *own* bodies feel and learn to put a name to these feelings? "If you're warm and tingly and you know it, then you're happy. If you're clenching your fists and you know it, then you're angry. If your heart is pumping hard and you know it, then you're scared." Being able to identify feelings in our bodies and name our own emotions seems a much better place to start.

Many of us are disconnected from our bodies. We are time-poor and sometimes register the sensations in our bodies only when they are big and overwhelming. But our interoceptive sense sends us hints constantly. The interoceptive receptors throughout our bodies pick up on the tiniest shifts and changes, but we rarely give these sensations any thought. When you take the time to check in on yourself, you become aware and can say "I am feeling…" The interoceptive sense is there to guide you on how you can best look after yourself. Do you need to sleep? Eat? Put on a sweater when the hairs rise on your skin?

Many autistic people process sensory information in a unique way, and the interoceptive sense is no exception. This sense of understanding how their bodies are feeling may be processed fast and furiously or not at all, or messages may be sent in a way that is confusing. For some people, body signals are so scrambled and vague that it is difficult to know where the feelings are coming from, or the feelings might be misinterpreted.

I have witnessed the confusion of body feelings in many autistic people. I have watched a young person fall from play equipment and, while in obvious pain from the fall, state through tears, "I'm hungry!" Of course, the child was not hungry but hurt. But the interoceptive sense of pain was unclear, and the mismatch of feeling in the brain brought forward the words of a different discomfort.

Jarrad was someone who had difficulty deciphering the signals his body sent him. He was a brilliant botanist who would dazzle me with his knowledge of plants' Latin names. He was attending university, and there, he had found "his people," others who could talk in plant language. Together, he and his classmates collected native Australian plant seeds to contribute to a seed bank. Jarrad was flourishing—in all but one thing.

Jarrad was frequently admitted to the hospital with uncontrollable panic attacks, and together we looked for the triggers that were causing them. Were they related to university and assignments? Deadlines and his need for perfection? Unexpected changes? Nope. They were related to heat. Jarrad had a panic attack if he was in an overheated room, if he had too many thick layers of clothing on, or if he sat in a car parked in the sun. Jarrad was not able to decipher the feelings within his body. His interoceptive sense was sending scrambled messages, and all "hot" feelings were quickly perceived as only one thing—panic.

Not everyone can process and clearly identify the sensations that the body is sending to the brain and give these feelings their correct emotional names. When we feel sad, our bodies may feel heavy, and when we're anxious, we may feel jittery. But how do we know how to interpret these body feelings? Some people (particularly those with alexithymia) really don't know how they feel and have trouble identifying and expressing their emotions.

We've all had times when we feel a certain way but are not sure why. *Why do I have this gnawing feeling? Why am I irritable? Why am I down in the dumps?* These feelings are clues, and taking note of these clues allows us to act.

A few years ago, a friend and I were walking through a farmers' market. The path was crowded with people, and the street was lined with parallel-parked cars. I was telling my friend something of little substance but of great interest to me: how juicy the strawberries that I had just bought were, or wondering aloud how people grow mushrooms. My friend and I were walking side by side when she suddenly quickened her pace and then broke into a run.

A child walking in an alley several paces in front of his parents had caught my friend's eye. In what seemed like a nanosecond, the child had run across the path and between the parked cars. My friend grabbed that child by the back of his jacket just as he was about to step into the road in front of a passing car. I felt the breeze of the car, heard the scream of the child's mother, and saw the flash of that red jacket as my friend pulled the child back just in time. I felt bile rise from my stomach as I thought about what could have happened. After thanks and tears from the parents, my friend and I continued on our way.

"How did you know?" I asked.

"I felt it in my gut" was all she said. "There were so many cars and kids, I felt something bad was about to happen. It was just a feeling."

Listening to our bodies and taking note of our interoceptive sense is the starting point of emotional fluency. We might be able to name hundreds of emotions, but if we don't actually know what each of these feels like, then having a huge vocabulary isn't helpful. We ask each other all the time, *How are you feeling?* But for many people, this is not an easily answered question.

And we can't ask this of others unless we can answer it for ourselves.

"It's hard to explain what a gut feeling is," I said to Margot, "and each person will feel it differently."

I told her that some people called it a sixth sense and that you felt it when your body sent you signals. It might be a churning in your stomach, a clamminess in your hands. You might become more aware and hypervigilant. Something in your head whispers, *This doesn't feel right.* And it is that whisper that you are meant to act on.

"In fact," I concluded, "it might feel like you're the passenger in a car with a bad driver, and you think you're about to crash."

Margot started to cry. Big wet tears rolled down her cheeks, and I could do nothing but watch her through the pixels of a screen six hundred miles away.

"My gut has been talking to me my whole life, but I wasn't listening," Margot said, sobbing. "My feelings are like a big tangled pile of Christmas lights that I wish I'd taken the time to untangle before putting them away for another year."

"You just didn't know the feeling in your body or have the language yet," I assured her.

We began to untangle the Christmas lights and she started to name her different bodily sensations.

"Sorrow is heavy and hollow," she said. "Sorrow is sticky tentacles wrapping around all your organs."

"And joy?" I asked her.

"Joy is a burst of bubbling energy. Your body feels warm and light. You feel like you're sparkling."

By creating a dictionary for the feelings of the body, Margot eventually became one of the most emotionally articulate people I know.

# 11

# Nikko's Rock

Sleeping in the same room with six teenage boys is not something I want to do every night of my life, but when you're a special-education teacher at a school camp, it's part of the job.

For many of the high-school students at camp, it was the first time they had slept away from home. There was a lot of homesickness, and the three nights felt like a lifetime. Every student was filled with trepidation, and they were all trying things for the first time: first time eating spaghetti Bolognese, first time sleeping in a sleeping bag, first time figuring out for themselves where their socks and undies were in the morning and where their pj's were at night. It was chaos. Everyone was nervous and there had been many tears from all of them— except Nikko.

Nikko looked like he meant business. He wore Metallica T-shirts and black jeans. He cut the sleeves from his shirts so they could show off his muscles, except he had no biceps to speak of. He was scrawny and slight and had the face of a waif, all protruding cheekbones and translucent skin.

Nikko always spoke with bravado. No matter what you'd done, he'd done it better. If you'd walked up a hill, Nikko had hiked up Mount Everest. If you had swum the length of an Olympic pool, Nikko had swum the English Channel.

We had lots of adventures at camp. We climbed trees, sang around campfires, toasted marshmallows, and caught tadpoles in the dam. Nikko announced his skills in climbing and lighting fires and shared his deep-sea fishing escapades with all who would listen.

One morning all of us went for a walk along a country road. We took many breaks, as one student was frightened by the sheep and cows and spent a lot of time crying and needing to sit down by the side of the road. Nikko became frustrated with the stopping and starting and began to complain about people being babies.

"Everyone gets scared, Nikko," I commented. "What are you scared of?"

"I'm not scared of anything," he said.

I knew that Nikko's bold assertion was not the whole truth. Anyone who boasted that much, who bragged that much, was usually hiding something.

And for Nikko, the truth was exposed by an eighteen-inch-high rock.

We all experience fear. Humans are hardwired to feel frightened, as it helps us avoid danger. It's an emotion that keeps us safe.

Most of us have a list of what we're scared of. Some are easily frightened by snakes, spiders, or rats. Some are afraid of flying, of visits to the dentist, or of heights. Some people fear events that haven't happened and might never happen, like losing their children, being kidnapped, becoming ill, or getting in a car accident. People fear the climate crisis, tsunamis, floods, and earthquakes. Some of these fears are logical, but others are created in our imaginations.

A dark bedroom at night is a breeding ground for irrational childhood fears. "I can't sleep," children cry. "There are ghosts and monsters in my room!" Darkness lights up the imagination. What is lurking in the corners? What could be hiding in the wardrobe or under the bed? Night-lights chase away the unknown, and it's in the unknown that danger exists. It's in the "what if" that many people's fears are based.

I have a friend who loves to swim, but not in the ocean. She will swim lap upon lap in a pool, because within those walls, she is safe from sharks. She's never actually encountered a shark, but each time she enters the water at the beach, she thinks she will.

"It's completely irrational," she told me, "but my imagination goes wild. I think sharks are everywhere. If a bit of seaweed even touches me, I scream."

I don't fear sharks; they never enter my thoughts. I do, however, sometimes think of giant squid, with their eyes as big as Frisbees and beaks strong enough to slice through a steel cable. When I'm in the water, I imagine their forty-foot-long tentacles wrapping around me and their suckers, with their little hooks, suctioning onto my skin. Yes, yes, I know that giant squid live in the deep, dark ocean, and I'm in water that's only up to my waist—but fear isn't always based in fact. And because I love the salt water, I have to tell myself that my fear is not real. But this isn't always easy to do.

Weylan was in his forties when he told me the story of the power lines. He had a PhD, worked as a researcher at the local university, and had published more journal articles than I had fingers and toes. He was a man of many words, but this hadn't always been the case; Weylan hadn't used words for the first six years of his life.

When he was a child, Weylan lived on a farm, and his

mother drove him through the countryside into town to attend speech therapy several times a week. He told me that he had recently driven the same road with his mom.

"Mom told me that I used to scream along that road," he said. "She asked if I could remember why. And of course I could. I was screaming about the power lines."

Weylan explained that there were large power lines along the road, the kind of huge high-voltage lines that carry electricity from the power plant into town. At one point, the wires crossed over the road, jumping from one pole to another.

"Every single time at that spot along the road, I'd look up at the wires through the windshield and think that they were going to fall on us," he remembered. "They looked like they would snap and hit the car."

At that age, he was nonspeaking, and Weylan hadn't been able to explain this fear to his mother, so she had no idea what was making him so upset. "Mom thought it was because I didn't like speech therapy—but I loved it," he said, "otherwise I never would have got into the car."

Motivation helps us push through fear. We'll do things that scare the hell out of us in order to feel the exhilaration of having done it, but we usually have to talk ourselves into it. One of the most common tools we have to overcome fear is self-talk.

We give ourselves our own personal pep talks. My neighbor Amber recently did the longest bungee jump in New Zealand. She showed me the video, but I was more interested in the footage of her *before* the jump than in the jump itself. She stood on a platform more than three hundred feet above a small pool of water, and everything in her body language screamed *I don't want to do it*. In the video, her teeth were clenched and her eyes darted about. She finally looked down and hid her face in her hands. She shook her head but shimmied slowly toward the edge. Once there, rather than standing up straight and bold, she squatted down.

"Do it, Amber. C'mon, Amber—just do it," she murmured to herself with conviction. And then, like a bolt of electricity had struck her, she stood and quickly dove off, headfirst, arms outstretched.

"It was thrilling," she recounted. "There's no feeling like it. But moving through the fear was one of the hardest things I've ever done."

Not everyone has the capacity to persevere through their feelings of fear. Convincing yourself to commit a death-defying stunt is one thing, but some people struggle to talk themselves into leaving the house, speaking up in meetings, or starting a conversation. Fear can stop people from participating in the simplest of everyday situations.

Many people love dogs, man's best friend. They can be great companions and give lots of love and affection, but they can also jump and lick and stink. At fifteen, Gaby had limited words, but one of her first had been *dog*. And not because she loved them. Gaby *hated* dogs.

While most teenagers love to take risks and test the boundaries, Gaby loved the safety of her own front yard—because outside that fence were dogs. If she left the yard, she always held her father's hand, and if she spotted a dog (even from hundreds of yards away), she would hide behind her father's back and scream and shake. It was impossible to take Gaby to the park; there were too many dogs. It was out of the question to go to the supermarket, as people tied their dogs up outside the doors. Gaby needed a lift to school every day, even though it was only two blocks away, because if she saw a dog along the way, she would run in the other direction.

One day, after Gaby's dads scouted the local beachside café

and saw no dogs in the vicinity, they managed to encourage Gaby to sit at a table for a milkshake. It was a big achievement for her, the first time she'd sipped a shake in a public place, but it lasted only minutes. Soon after, a couple arrived and sat down at a table...with their dog. They were only a few feet away, and Gaby, seeing the fluffy golden retriever, reacted in sheer horror and climbed onto the table. Once up there, she refused to come down until the dog was no longer in sight.

Many autistic people experience emotions intensely. Magnify your feeling of fear, and you might approach the terror that they can feel. I've known autistic people who are terrified of balloons, horrified by grass, or scared to death of blenders and vacuums. For Gaby, it was dogs.

When an autistic person is petrified, neurological pathways can become paralyzed too. When people feel the sensations of fear, their brains can become so overwhelmed that they are unable to think clearly. They can't hear the calming thoughts that come with self-talk. What's worse, others sometimes minimize whatever it is that is frightening them. To Gaby, it wasn't "just a dog"—it was an immediate threat.

"It's difficult explaining to dog lovers that Gaby is petrified," one of her fathers told me. "And we don't even understand why. She's never been bitten. Maybe it's that dogs are so unpredictable, and Gaby loves predictability."

Fear can be based on unpredictability. We all want to know what is going to happen next, and when we don't know what the outcome of a situation will be, our thoughts can go wild. We imagine everything that will go wrong and conjure up scenes of pain and suffering. And it's only natural that we try to avoid what will hurt us, even if it exists only in our imaginations. We all back away from things that are bad, like rotting food and spiders' webs. We're also motivated by reward and want to move toward the things that we love, like cake and the smell of garde-nias. As humans, we are designed to move toward the good and away from the bad, and this also applies to our emotions.

Excitement and happiness are considered "good" emotions; uncertainty and sadness are "bad." But emotions shouldn't be labeled like this. All emotions serve a purpose and each has an important role to play in our lives. Fear is not "bad." We need fear. Fear is a warning signal to be on guard. We need to listen to our bodies and know when to be on the alert. Fear says, *Don't get too close to the edge.*

Fear also gives us the adrenaline to help us through diffi-cult moments. Have you ever done something that was really hard, something that you are really proud you did? Gotten your driver's license, done well on an exam, played in a champi-onship with your team? When we're moving toward a goal and want to succeed, we often begin to feel frightened. This fear says, *I really want to do well at this* or *This is important to me.* It's the fear of failure, the fear that we won't do our best when we so desperately want to. But we don't always recognize these feelings as good for us.

People who have difficulty interpreting the sensations and feelings in their bodies, especially if they're neurodivergent, can have a hard time differentiating between the kind of fear that warns of danger and the kind people feel because they want to succeed. They can fear *fear* itself and will avoid any activity that causes it.

When we're frightened, when we back away from what scares us, we need encouragement. The word *encouragement* lit-erally means "to put courage in." When we support one another by building each other's confidence, we build courage. We can help each other take the leap, risk it, show up, give it a go, or even just hold on.

Being courageous isn't about *not* feeling fear. In fact, it's fear that makes us brave. True courage comes when you are shaking in your boots, your stomach is tied in knots, and every cell in your body is screaming *No way, don't do it!*—and you do it anyway. People aren't courageous only when they fight fires or dive into rapid rivers—they can also be courageous when they get a blood test, ride a roller coaster, carry a bug outside, or swim in an ocean full of squid the length of shipping containers.

When people can't hear their own thoughts over the roar of fear, others need to whisper quietly or scream loudly to them, *Keep trying. It's okay. You can do it!*

According to Nikko, he'd been in base camp in the Himalayas, but this wasn't apparent on the day we went to the beach. We wandered down a track that sloped toward the ocean and ended at a rock. This rock wasn't hanging from the side of a cliff or anything—it was about the height of a rolling pin and cushioned with soft sand below.

The students walked one behind the other along the path, each of them stepping down off the rock in stride. Then it was Nikko's turn.

Nikko looked down and I saw his eyes widen and the veins in his skinny neck bulge. Then he froze, not a muscle moving, with a grimace of fear plastered on his color-drained face.

"Come on, Nikko," I said. "It's just one small step."

But I might as well have asked him to jump from a plane. He staggered a few steps back and then moved forward again. What I saw as a shin-high step down, Nikko perceived as a gulf-like chasm. This step turned his legs to jelly, and it was impossible for him to move.

"No, no, no," he repeated over and over again.

Then one child called out, "You can do it, Nikko!" and

other students began to chant like a crowd at a football match. This surprised me. Nikko had spent the past two days letting everyone know what he thought of their fears—"Only a wuss won't eat spag Bol," "You're a chicken," "It's only a sleeping bag"—but no one called Nikko a scaredy-cat. No one put him down; they just encouraged him to step down.

The students called his name again and again in a chorus of support: "Nikko, Nikko, Nikko!"

Quietly, he began to talk to himself. He stepped out of his own body and became his own encouraging bystander. "It's okay, Nikko," he muttered. "You can do it, Nikko."

It took every ounce of courage he could muster. He raised his chin, stood tall, and pushed his shoulders back. For a moment he was motionless, unwavering.

"*Do it, Nikko!*" he suddenly yelled. And with his eyes closed, he stepped into his unknown.

# 12

# Ellis's Three Days

Ellis likes rules, and he likes *everyone* to follow the rules. If you're driving when Ellis is on the road, you better be on your best behavior. If Ellis spots you breaking the road rules, he will take down your license-plate number and call the police.

During the years of the pandemic, rules were everywhere: lockdowns, masks, six feet between people, and standing on designated spots. Ellis, who worked in an office, asked if his boss could guarantee that all employees would wear masks and sit in their assigned spaces with the required distance between them.

"We're trying, Ellis," his boss assured him. "We're following the requirements that allow us to return to work, but I cannot one hundred percent tell you that all employees will keep their required distance and consistently wear their masks appropriately."

"Don't tell me that!" Ellis said sternly. "I'll need to report you. I will need to call the COVID hotline if the organization cannot do exactly what it is expected to do!"

After that, Ellis did not return to his job at the office for weeks. He waited until all restrictions had eased and went back only when he was certain that everyone would be able to do *exactly* what was expected of them.

"Why are rules so important, Ellis?" I asked.

"Because rules are established to look after us," he said. "If you use your phone when driving or don't sanitize your hands, you obviously don't care if you hurt other people. Rule-breakers only think about themselves." Ellis was the social-justice police, and for him rules were *not* meant to be broken.

One day, Ellis casually said, "My father died two weeks ago."

"Oh my God, Ellis, I'm so sorry," I said. "I can't imagine how hard that must be."

"It's okay, I'm fine now," he said. "That was two weeks ago. I was sad for the three days that we are allowed to be sad for."

"Three days?" I said in a wave of confusion. "What do you mean, three days?"

"That's our allocated bereavement leave in our work contracts," he stated simply. "According to the rules, we're allowed three days to grieve, so I felt sad for the seventy-two hours assigned."

Ellis followed the regulations; he didn't jaywalk and he didn't litter. He diligently complied with the laws requiring him to wear a seat belt and pay his taxes on time. But surely there were no rules when it came to grief?

We all experience loss. Sadly, it's part of being human.

Some losses are slight and some are staggering. We lose races, coming in second or last; we lose favorite toys or valued pieces of jewelry. We experience the loss of jobs, friendships, relationships, and pets. Every loss brings sadness. We feel that all is not right with the world, and it takes time to right ourselves again.

And then there is the ultimate loss: losing the people we love.

The heart represents love. As a teenager, depending on my emotional state, I covered books with drawings of plump red hearts, hearts with Cupid's arrows punched through them, and hearts cracking in two. When I drew those broken hearts, I never really understood why they had fault lines like tectonic plates. I didn't realize that a broken heart felt like an earthquake that shook you to your core.

Then Maria died.

Maria and I were like Shrek and Donkey. We were complete opposites, but she could peel back all the layers of my onion. She was the most loyal and trusted of friends. We're lucky to have these kinds of people in our lives, the people we turn to when the shit hits the fan, the ones who make us believe we are capable of battling dragons. When we're shattered, they gather us close with wide-open arms, with no judgment. When we succeed, they pop the champagne (although my Maria hated champagne). Even on an ordinary day, when we see something special or learn something new, we want to share that with them.

Maria was one of those people. She was my person.

A few years ago, Maria was diagnosed with cancer. Her cancer's name is not one you'd recognize because it is so aggressive there is little time for research. It does not have a "day" or a ribbon. It is a cancer that is brutal and cruel.

Maria was full of life, and then over just a few short months, all that life was taken away.

And then she was gone ... just gone.

It was in grieving Maria that I understood why the emotion is called a broken heart: because your heart feels like it has detonated into pieces. It's pulverized. I could feel it and had to grab at my chest and press down hard to keep it from exploding out onto the floor.

Grief is visceral. It attacks every part of you, your thoughts and your feelings. It bleeds into every nerve and sinew. It invades your muscles and bones. It takes away your appetite and your sleep. It robs you of your concentration, your short-term memory, your ability to hear, listen, and connect with others. Emotions that you never knew existed raise their heads and roar and wail.

Grief is both psychological and physical. Grief can cause depression, anger, guilt, and hopelessness. When you're grieving, the brain releases massive amounts of hormones and chemicals that change the way your body functions. Grief changes all of us, but the way grief is felt, the way it is experienced, and the way it presents is vastly different for everyone.

When I was working as an outreach teacher to support the inclusion of students with disabilities in mainstream schools, I received a phone call: Sean was urinating in the classroom. Sean was defecating in his pants. Sean had not done this since he was toilet-trained at five years old, but he was doing it now at thirteen. Something was not right.

Sean was a giggler. He loved sticks and gathered them whenever he was outdoors. He had an impressive collection. He didn't like solid sticks with no bend in them, though; they were discarded, sent back to the ground's bargain basement. Sean liked new-growth, bendy green sticks that swished with the sound of a basketball shooting through the net or a silk dress against your legs as you walk. With every swish, Sean giggled.

Sean didn't speak, but he expressed himself in grunts, hums, teeth-grinding, and laughter. He had a communication system to indicate yes or no, make basic food choices, and request to stay inside or go out. He communicated most of his wants and needs by actions. If he didn't want to participate, he would walk away. If he wanted something from the top shelf, he would climb up to it.

Now Sean was trying to say something.

"So has something happened at school?" I asked the staff member. "Any changes? Anything new?"

"No, nothing."

"No renovations? New paint? New carpet? New teachers? New students? Change in routine?"

"Nothing."

"When did this start?"

"Oh, a few months ago. Maybe five?"

"Any changes at home then? Anything that he could be trying to tell us?"

"Well, his mom died about six months ago," the teacher's aide said. "But Sean doesn't even know what day of the week it is. He has no idea what's happening in the world around him and he wouldn't have any understanding of death. And anyway, that was months ago."

My mind went somewhere dark. Even though I had never done it, I imagined what it would feel like to punch someone in the face.

Sean's mother had died. She was here and then she was not.

Sean's mom had been his everything. She was the person he opened his eyes to in the morning. She was the hand in his when a dog was in sight; she was the singer in the bathroom when the shampoo hurt his eyes; she was the patter of the towel to dry him. She was the passer of the correct seamless socks and the counter of buttons one by one from top to bottom on his shirts. She was the ham-and-cheese-sandwich-cut-into-four-triangles-with-no-crust-maker; the voice of Homer, Marge, Bart, and Lisa when things were hard; and the scratcher of his head to put him to sleep at night. And then she was no more.

Sean's mom had disappeared and never returned.

"So you are telling me that nothing—not a *single thing*—has changed that would make this kid feel so lost, hurt, and confused that he would wet and shit himself?" I seethed. For me, this was beyond belief.

Loss in all its forms is complex for everyone. Some people may have intense immediate reactions; for others, grief may be delayed for days, weeks, or months. There is no typical response when it comes to grief, no textbook grieving process. We all grieve in our own way, and we should never judge the grieving process of others. We just need to be there for anyone experiencing its turmoil.

The way neurodivergent people express grief can sometimes be viewed as a behavior associated with autism rather than just a natural expression of loss. Some autistic people have difficulty processing their feelings or might not show their distress through the expected gestures. They might not display any outward emotions; they might not cry or weep or appear sad; their demeanor might not change. Their behavior might be interpreted as being unfeeling, but this is simply untrue—they just might feel in a different way.

Autistic people might have increased hypersensitivity or more meltdowns; they might withdraw or become clingy and experience separation anxiety. Some might not show any response for months, and then their delayed distress might be misunderstood and seen as a reaction to something altogether different. An autistic person might not have the ability to communicate, months after a death, the feeling of "I'm curled into a ball and crying right now because I just smelled the lavender talcum powder my grandma wore, and I'm missing her."

Some autistic people become stuck trying to make sense of it all, and they ask the same questions over and over: "So, Nan is buried? What happens to the body? Why did she die?" This can be viewed as insensitive, but death leaves all of us with unanswerable questions. The way that we discuss death and dying can create even more confusion for some autistic people, who require simple and clear information presented in a way that they can comprehend. Telling an autistic person that someone has "gone to sleep" basically means the person will wake up. Or take the expression *passed away*. What does *pass away* even mean? By avoiding the truth—not saying the word *died*—we add to the uncertainty and misunderstanding of death, particularly for people who just need the plain facts.

Grief hits all of us in waves and in rolling sets. We are smashed, pummeled, and dumped, turned upside down and inside out. Then, slowly but surely, though we may still feel lost at sea, with the passing of the sun and the seasons and the turning of the calendar from one year to the next, we arrive in calmer waters. We will all feel it, but for each of us, the reaction to the breaking swell will be different.

"What was that three days like for you, Ellis?" I asked.

Ellis told me that he didn't know what grieving was. No one he knew had ever died before. He'd never owned a goldfish or a hamster or a cat. He had never known that after death comes a period of mourning. No one had ever talked with Ellis about death or grief.

He didn't know what he was meant to do, and he wanted to follow the rules—so he'd looked it up. The internet told him that there are stages of grief. Ellis viewed these as linear steps he was to follow: shock, denial, anger, bargaining, depression, acceptance, and processing.

"I wrote up a timetable to get through all the stages in the three days," he explained. "But I didn't go through them all. I didn't get angry and I didn't deny. Dad's dead—there's no denying that. I was sad, but I'm not sad anymore."

It sounded so clinical, so detached, yet my heart felt so heavy. Ellis might not have been sad anymore, but I was sad for him. I wished so much that grief could be squashed into a clear timetable so we knew when it would end—that there was an end in sight. But it couldn't be, and I knew it. I knew that Ellis's grief timetable held no box where he could tick off *Completed*.

"What have you been up to in the last two weeks, then?" I asked. "Are you back at work?"

"Of course, that is what I wanted to discuss with you," he said. "My work hasn't been good."

Ellis told me that he was normally excellent at his job but he had been making lots of mistakes. He felt he couldn't process the information properly, and his boss had found his errors.

"Maybe it's because I'm having trouble sleeping?" he wondered aloud. "I have insomnia and am awake most of the night. And I think I'm getting sick too; I might be getting a cold. I've had a headache for days now. It's right behind my eyes and down the back of my neck. Do you think I have caught a virus, Jodi?"

Grief is like a virus; it enters your body and mind and plays havoc with them. It flattens you, stabs at you, and creates aches and pains—but it doesn't leave you. Grief layers itself under your skin and settles there. It continues to shift from being buried deep down to sitting just below the surface. And it appears again and again, sometimes in emptiness, sometimes in disbelief, sometimes in tears, and sometimes in the laughter of wonderful memories.

Grief has no rules and it has no time limit. The intensity of loss does subside, but we never fully recover.

The scars of having loved always remain.

### PART II

# Sharing Our Point of View

Expressing and Understanding

In the 1990s, full of wanderlust and seeking adventure, I moved to Southeast Asia. These were the days before mobile phones and the internet, and my contact with home was through handwritten letters picked up at the poste restante every two months.

For almost two years, I lived on a remote island 0.4 degrees from the equator. It was a three-boat trip to get there from Singapore, each boat getting smaller and less comfortable. The final leg of the journey was all diesel fumes and motion sickness. This island was not on the tourist route, and there were no full-moon parties to entice backpackers. A travel guidebook (which was our 1990s Tripadvisor) stated that "the fish and vegetable markets near the harbor are interesting to wander around." That was the island's main—and only—attraction.

When I first arrived, I experienced culture shock. The customs were completely unknown to me. I didn't understand the religion or the etiquette of dress. I couldn't understand what people were saying. I didn't get their sense of humor, and I kept getting the rules wrong for how to be courteous and polite. I didn't know that I was supposed to lower my body below the faces of two people talking and extend my right hand in front of me when I walked between them. I didn't know that when greeting others, I was supposed to raise both of my hands to my heart, that I should give or accept something only with my right hand, and that showing the soles of my feet was disrespectful.

Arriving in a foreign country where you don't understand the spoken language or the body language or the culture or any of the customs is terrifying. I was a white, non-Muslim

English-speaker living in a community of Asian, Muslim non-English-speakers. I had no idea what I was doing or how to fit in. It was exhausting.

On waking, I would go over the routine of my day in my head. I'd practice the words I'd need in social situations. I would run through the scripts of these yet-to-happen interactions: how I would carry my body, how I would dress, and what would be appropriate to say and do in terms of my gender in this community. I came to rely on these words and scripts and routines.

Each morning I headed to the market to buy what was needed for the day. I had lists of words for the vegetables and fruit, and I would repeat them to myself over and over. It was difficult at first because I didn't understand the people at the market, and they didn't understand me. I was shy and embarrassed, slow in understanding and slower in speaking. But at the market, I found someone who had the patience to show me each vegetable and fruit in turn and repeat the words for me so I could get the sounds right. And this person became part of my routine.

Every day, I headed to the same stall and the same person who sat among the carrots, tempeh, and jackfruit. And with each visit, my anxiety lifted, just a little.

In the early days, after I went to this one stall, I needed to go somewhere quiet, somewhere I could be alone so I could think of my next list of words and the next script for the day. But as my confidence grew, I would venture out a little farther, maybe to one more shop or to the coffeehouse or to buy some fried noodles. Although I still tired easily from these simple interactions and the amount of brainpower it took for me to communicate, these connections gave me great joy.

So I tried hard to learn. Learn the language. Learn the

culture. Learn the customs. Learn how to communicate. I attempted to fill the chasm I felt between myself and others.

But this community of people did not expect me to know. They didn't expect me to "become" them. They didn't expect me to speak the language correctly, and they didn't rush me or laugh at me. When I was doing something culturally inappropriate, they explained it to me. They didn't shun me or chastise me. They took their time and sat with me, slowly repeating words and showing me gestures. And within these beautiful exchanges, over time, I knew that my difference was just as wonderful to them as theirs was to me.

I was different, but I learned that being different was just fine. It was fine because the people around me accepted these differences and tried to communicate with me as much as I tried to communicate with them.

People use words, gestures, facial expressions, or a combination of all three to communicate our wants and needs, our thoughts and emotions. But we also have to be receptive to what is being communicated. We have to listen, see, understand, and comprehend. We're not always clear in the way we express ourselves, and sometimes we can misunderstand what another person is trying to convey. Of course, neurotypical people experience miscommunication; I'm sure that you can think of countless examples when what was said differed from what was understood. Many autistic people experience this kind of misunderstanding in every social interaction. Autistic people may express themselves differently and have difficulty interpreting what is being communicated. It can seem as though neurodivergent and neurotypical people speak completely different languages.

If you really want to know what that feels like, travel to a place where you don't know the language or the customs or the culture, and you will begin to understand how complex and difficult this can be—how *exhausting* it is. This is the experience of many autistic people every single day.

During my time in Indonesia, I learned how difficult it was to communicate, and this was one of the greatest gifts I have ever received. Throughout my career, it has reminded me how important it is to develop deeper empathy and connection with people who are different from myself. It has helped me shed all my preconceived ideas, let go of my point of view, and move toward people with their own way of communicating and interacting.

We all need people in our lives who can help us make sense of the world. We need our own vegetable-stall owner on a remote island with a little time and a lot of patience. We need to help one another out with translation.

# 13

# Jonathan's Eleven

S orry, sorry, sorry," Jonathan said every time he and his family walked down a crowded street. He said it to no one in particular, and his parents had no idea why.

When I met the family, Jonathan was a quiet, shy ten-year-old who always carried a calculator, pen, and notepad with him. He loved numbers and sums, and he was good at all things numerical. In fact, he was doing brilliantly in math and was working on the high-school math curriculum while in the fourth grade. He might have been clumsy and uncoordinated, and he hated gym class, but he could recite the players on every basketball team and their stats by heart. (The phys ed teacher loved this, which gave him an advantage in other ways.)

Jonathan had received an autism diagnosis just eighteen months before. The pediatrician had given his parents a letter stating this fact and sent the family on their way, which left them unsure about what this meant for Jonathan or how they could best support him. Jonathan's parents were struggling to understand both their son and each other. The most easily accessible information Jonathan's parents had was Google, and we all know the rabbit holes Dr. Google can send you down.

You only have to type in *autism* to be lost in there for days. And Google wasn't giving Jonathan's parents the answers they needed. It wasn't answering their *big* question: why would Jonathan follow instructions only if they were given by his father?

We all make requests of children: "Pick up your wet towel." "Put your bowl in the sink." "Put your toys away." We expect that by the time children reach a certain age, they will participate in the household chores. Jonathan's parents were no exception; after all, Jonathan was ten.

"He won't do anything I ask," his mom lamented when she and her husband came to see me on their own. "I give Jonathan an instruction and he ignores me. I ask and ask. Repeating myself like this drives me mad. I get frustrated and can even get a little hot under the collar with him. He will not do *a thing* for me, but my husband just has to ask once or twice and he does it straightaway!"

Sometimes, trying to figure out how an autistic person perceives the world is like trying to solve a mystery. The first step is simply to ask why someone does what they do. I asked Jonathan why he followed instructions from Dad and not from Mom.

"Dad gets angry but Mom is never angry," he said. "I know she's never angry because she doesn't have an eleven!"

"An eleven? What does that mean?" I pondered, scrunching up my nose and a corner of my mouth in response.

We communicate *a lot* with our faces. That small space has forty-three muscles, and they are contracted and expanded in various combinations to express feelings and thoughts. All cultures of the world recognize the facial expressions for sixteen emotions. Give it a go—turn the volume down next time you're watching a movie and see if you can recognize anger, amusement, awe, concentration, confusion, contempt, contentment, desire, disappointment, doubt, elation, interest, pain, sadness, surprise, and triumph on the faces on the screen.

Facial expressions generally last for up to four seconds, so most people can get a good look at them and easily understand how the other person is feeling. Many young children can tell you when someone is happy, sad, or scared by the distinct manner in which faces demonstrate these emotions.

But we also have micro-expressions, which can be as brief as half a second. It's in these moments that our true emotions appear and any mismatch between our thoughts and feelings can be seen. Reading these fleeting expressions takes a level of skill. Many of us, neurotypical and neurodivergent alike, might not register these movements, might misread them, or might not understand their meaning.

It is commonly believed that autistic people have great difficulty reading facial expressions, but this is not altogether true. Many autistic people are able to read the main facial expressions because they're fairly consistent across all human faces, and they stick around long enough for people to see them. It's the millisecond nuance of the micro-expression that can be complicated to discern, and therein lies the difficulty.

Think of how clever people are with their expressions, how they sometimes show one thing but feel another. For instance, when you smile and feign gratitude on receiving a crap gift.

I can be terrible at giving presents, so I'm regularly on the receiving end of this forced smile. Not long ago, I bought someone I cherish a gift, and I was thrilled with myself because I thought I had gotten it just right. The person opened it, smiled graciously, and said, "Oh, thank you, it's brilliant." But I saw it: the confusion. It was slight and fleeting, but it said, *Why the hell has she given me this?* If I'd missed that half-second flinch, I would still be congratulating myself on my supreme shopping abilities.

When I gave a birthday gift to an autistic friend a few years ago, she didn't shy away from the truth or pretend in any way. She just said, "Jodi, I hate this." I loved the honesty. When the same friend looked completely nonchalant at my gift the following year but said, "I love it," I knew it was true, even though I didn't see any facial expression indicating appreciation.

While most people recognize the universal facial expressions, these expressions can convey very different emotions depending on the context. A person needs to be able to take into account the context in which these expressions are being used, otherwise the intent behind the expression can be misinterpreted. A smile can mean many things depending on when and how it is used.

Did you know that there are nineteen different types of smiles but only six actually express happiness? We can smile when we're embarrassed or horrified or in pain, although I'm not sure that "grinning and bearing it" is the best use of our smiles. Smiles can be contagious when they convey happiness, but not all smiles truly express joy.

Recently I was staying with someone who knows me very, very well. I was on my way to the kitchen to wash some dishes while he was watching his all-time-favorite cooking show. As I passed, I turned to him and smiled.

"That is the fakest smile I've ever seen you do," he said. "It was completely plastic."

"How'd you know?" I asked, because he was right. I was just throwing a smile *at* him; it was not a genuine smile *for* him.

"Because that smile never reached your eyes," he said. He could see right through me.

While we all get away with fake smiles every now and then, we sometimes mistake one type of smile for another. Not being able to read a smile for what it is truly expressing can cause problems.

"He never takes us seriously," Isaac's mom told me over the phone before I met her son. "He thinks everything we say is a complete joke. He's been in trouble with the police and is at risk of being expelled from school, but whenever we try to discipline him, he just smirks at us. It's infuriating."

Isaac was intimidating. He was a beefy eighteen-year-old with a crew cut and a death stare. In one hand he carried a coin that he rolled between his fingers with incredible dexterity. After seeing this trick performed by Jack Sparrow in *Pirates of the Caribbean,* Isaac had spent months and months mastering the knuckle roll. But it wasn't his sleight of hand that commanded attention; it was his "smile," which conveyed bold, pompous confidence.

Isaac's smirk, which is imprinted on my brain, was smug and stiff. It took a long time for me to see the other side of Isaac — that he was a very funny guy. He had a repertoire of dad jokes with terrible punch lines, and I would giggle and groan every time he told one. But if I had gone on my first impression, I would never have seen this Isaac. I wouldn't have seen him because his smirk was so full of arrogance that I would have viewed him as only condescending and patronizing.

But Isaac's smirk was always strained and clenched. I could tell that something wasn't quite right because the same expression would appear each and every time we talked about the hard stuff — the stuff that was getting him into such big trouble.

"Isaac, when you grin like this," I said, showing him with my own face, "what are you feeling?"

"Scared," he said. "My face does this when I'm nervous."

A nervous smile can look like a smirk. Because he was anxious, Isaac couldn't wipe the grin off his face as his parents asked him to do when they scolded him. We'd all been reading Isaac's face wrong. We needed to see his smirk for what it really was: anxiety.

Some people, like Isaac, have their expressions misread, while others show little to no facial expression at all.

Dean had a stoic face and an attitude toward life that matched. He was unflappable. If you wanted to know about minimalism, how to live a life of nonconsumption, or how to make every single cent work for you, Dean was your man.

At thirty-four years old, Dean didn't believe in using energy that wasn't renewable. He had never had a driver's license and traveled only by bike. He had studied the minimum number of calories a person needed to consume to stay healthy, and he ate only the appropriate amount of vegetables, fruit, fat, grains, and protein daily. He had studied native foods, could light a fire without flint, and religiously kept his first aid certificate up-to-date.

As a counselor, you spend most of your time with clients considering their facial expressions. In the game of poker, everyone has a "tell," a subtle and slight change in demeanor that gives you a clue as to what's in that person's hand. With clients, you're watching for those micro-expressions that provide insight into their thoughts and feelings.

Dean had a poker face, and he had no tell. He never furrowed his brow or showed his crow's-feet. His face was still and unmoving. This is known as a "flat affect." When I am joyful, I have a wide-open smile that shows the fillings in my back molars. When Dean was joyful, his face was neutral. When I am horrified, my mouth gapes open and my eyes bulge. When Dean was horrified, his face was neutral. When I am gripped with sadness, my eyes are cast down and the corners of my lips follow. When Dean was sad, his face was neutral. We expect others to register emotions on their faces, but Dean's emotions were hidden.

And while I couldn't read Dean's face, he also couldn't read mine. "Are you angry with me?" "Did you think that was funny?" "Did that make you sad?" Dean checked in with me constantly when we were together for appointments. He would tell me a story but could not understand how I felt about it from my facial expressions. If I was listening intently, eyes lowered, he would think I was upset. If I was concerned and wrinkled my eyebrows, Dean would think that I was sad. Dean could not judge a book by its cover.

"People call me rude," Dean told me. "Sometimes they say I am stuck-up or that I am ungrateful. Others tell me that I am unfeeling...that hurts. Just because my face doesn't work the same as theirs, I'm not any of those things. I feel too."

We can't assume that every smile means someone is happy or that a blank face means the opposite. We also can't assume that similar expressions on two people's faces are conveying the same emotion or that two different expressions don't mean the same thing. People's facial movements convey what they are feeling and thinking, but when there are so many variations in expressions, so many momentary, transient shifts, it's a wonder any of us can understand each other at all.

And what about Jonathan's eleven?

To better understand the many facial expressions people displayed, Jonathan had devised a unique numbering system for each one.

"Dad gets angry when he asks me to do a chore, so I do it," he told me. "Mom is never angry, so when she asks me to do something and I don't do it, she really doesn't care that much."

Jonathan had labeled his dad's angry face 11, because when his father was frustrated, he would knit his eyebrows together, creating two deep lines between his brows. His mom, however, was still and stony-faced in expressing her anger. Because she didn't have an 11 between her brows, Jonathan assumed she wasn't serious about her requests, so he would just ignore them.

Jonathan's number code also explained his constant apologizing to strangers. When I asked him why he said "Sorry" to everyone while he was walking down the street, he said that he didn't apologize to everyone—just the angry 11s. "Most of them are old and have wrinkles," he said, "but they all have an eleven, so I figure I must have done something to upset them!"

Jonathan's parents were astonished that Jonathan had developed a coded system for emotions but also that he viewed their expressions of the same emotion so differently. Jonathan taught them more of his system. Surprise was a 0, because that was the shape the mouth made. Scared was 000, because that was the shape of the eyes *and* the mouth. Excitement was 3, because a 3 on its side was his mom's face when she was happy: "It's your smile and two dimples," he told her. After learning the system, Jonathan's mom and dad used his code to name their emotions with him.

"Jonathan, I'm getting to an eleven now, I'm upset and angry," his perfectly smooth-faced (but still irritated) mother now said.

And with that Jonathan would pick up his wet towel from his carpeted bedroom floor.

# 14

# Dennis's Nod

I just can't put my finger on it," Dennis's teacher said. "Dennis looks like he's not interested, but he's obviously taking it in because he gets top marks on his tests. He just shows *no* enthusiasm or attention in class at all."

When I worked as a resource teacher in a large high school, my job was to help the mainstream teaching staff be inclusive in their teaching practices and modify their lesson plans to support the learning of neurodivergent kids.

When I first saw Dennis, he was sitting in a classroom full of boys. He reminded me of a whippet: he was sinewy and wiry, and his head looked too big for his lean body. He had large, protruding eyes that were magnified by bottle-thick reading glasses. Dennis was smart. He was getting top grades at school in math and science and had received academic awards at the end of each high-school year so far.

The students in his class were rowdy, and there was that distinct combination of low and deep voices interspersed with cracks of high-pitched squeaks that you hear in groups of boys in mid-puberty. Dennis wasn't engaged in the antics of the other pupils, though, nor did he show any interest in what the teacher at the front of the class was saying. He was sitting quietly on one side of the classroom, head resting in his hand, gazing out the window.

Dennis and I met after class so that I could try to gauge his ability to interact socially. I asked him a few questions and he told me he loved biology and that he'd dissected a cow's eye in science class the day before. "Wow, things haven't changed," I said, and I shared my memories of dissecting cows' hearts and cutting up frogs decades earlier.

For a moment I thought that Dennis wasn't interested in what I was saying. And then the light bulb went off in my head. He looked like he wasn't interested because he didn't use typical body language.

Dennis wasn't nodding his head.

When I'm giving a presentation to an auditorium full of people, I always survey the room. I scan the hundred-odd faces in front of me in search of feedback. I'm looking to see if anyone is sleeping (if I'm unlucky) or smiling and laughing (if I'm lucky), but mostly I am looking for the nod. I am looking for the body language that says, *Yes, I understand. Yes, that makes sense. Yes, keep talking.*

People nod their heads to encourage others to continue speaking. Nodding demonstrates that you are engaged in what is being said. Try this next time you're talking with people: tell them a story about your day (making sure they're not distracted by other things) and see how often they nod their heads. They won't even know they're doing it.

We're not taught to nod. No one ever sat a child down and said, "Nod your head when another person is talking so that they know you are listening." We just do it. When babies first start babbling, caregivers will pretend to hold a conversation with them, nodding at the babies' gibberish to motivate them to keep going. We do this to babies because people have been nodding at us since *we* were babies. This nodding gave us a sense of confidence, so we nod at the next generation to give them confidence too.

We communicate using our bodies from as early as three months of age. Babies will rub their eyes when tired and wriggle their arms and legs when excited. In these first years of life, a neurotypical child starts developing a range of nonverbal social-interaction skills by mimicking others. Many autistic children, however, aren't wired to watch and copy what other people do, and sometimes they interpret gestures in unique ways. For example, waving. When people wave hello or goodbye, they usually show the palms of their hands. I have witnessed young autistic children copy the waving gesture, but instead of presenting their palms to another person, they wave backward, with their palms facing themselves. It makes complete sense, really, as they are reflecting exactly what the other person is doing.

We use our bodies to communicate and respond to countless gestures every day. Our bodies reinforce the meaning behind our words as well as communicate emotion and intent. People direct their legs toward a person they are having a conversation with to show engagement; fold their arms to demonstrate displeasure or defensiveness; and shrug their shoulders to indicate *I don't know.* They lean in to express interest and pinch the bridge of the nose when confused. They signal with their hands, rub their fingers together to indicate money, kiss the ends of their fingers to signify *Delicious,* and turn their thumbs down for bad and up for good. We're not taught these nonverbal gestures the same way we're taught the letters of the alphabet. Using gestures comes naturally to the majority of neurotypical people; they pick it up as they go, and it's done without any conscious thought. When they communicate, their bodies just get in on the act.

Maeve didn't use any of these gestures. Even though she was thoughtful and generous, she had come to see me for support in developing relationships. I once mentioned I liked early-morning ocean swims, and the next session she brought me a printed table of that month's tides. She always offered to share her muffin with me and often came into my office with bunches of handpicked lavender. If Maeve's body language had matched her generosity, her physical expression would have been open and flowing; instead, her body was more like a mannequin in a shop window. Her movements were robotic, precise, and halting. Maeve did not talk with her hands; they were superglued to her sides.

"Have you heard of body language?" I once asked her.

"Body language?" She snorted. "Bodies don't have a language!"

I asked her if she had ever played charades. When she said no, I downloaded an app so that we could play together. "You can't speak, though," I explained. "You can't have any words come out of your mouth. In one minute, you have to use your body to communicate as many words as you can."

I had the first go. The app gave me *bow and arrow, hammering, making a sandwich, pogo stick,* and *playing catch.* I wasn't great, and Maeve missed some.

Then it was Maeve's turn; she got *juggling, taking a photo, gargling, playing violin, tying shoelaces,* and *sleepwalking.* I understood every single thing that she tried to convey to me, everything that her body was saying. Maeve was a master of mime.

"Oh, I get it," she said. "Bodies talk."

Different cultures have their own unique body language,

passed from one generation to the next. Some gestures are universal across cultures, but others have different meanings depending on where you are. A specific gesture may be perfectly fine in one culture but a sign of disrespect in another. Holding up two fingers can indicate the number 2, peace, victory, or *Up yours.* When you're trying to get someone to come over to you, do you signal with the palm up and one beckoning finger (as in the United States) or the palm down (as in Japan)? When you meet a friend, do you shake hands, not touch at all, or kiss on the cheek once (Philippines), twice (Italy), or three times (Switzerland)? Pointing is also particularly, well, *pointy.* "It's rude to point" is a rule linked to this gesture, since pointing directly at people can be viewed as threatening and aggressive. The finger that's used to point also differs depending on which country you are in, and if you are in Papua New Guinea, the nose is used instead of the finger.

No matter what appendage you use, pointing is a particularly powerful gesture that is learned early. Children learn to point before they can talk, but at no time does anyone take a child's hand and curl back all but the index finger to show how it's done. No, children watch caregivers point to pictures in books and the world around them, then they copy this gesture to make requests and statements without words.

I used to chat with my neighbor as she carried her baby around the garden. Watching him learn to communicate in his first year was wonderful. He would see a butterfly or a passing plane, jiggle up and down in her arms, and point. I would watch as my neighbor looked over to where he indicated, and through his gestures, I could almost hear him say, *How cool is that!* We don't need speech to communicate in such a dynamic way.

Pointing is an early developing social skill known as "joint attention." Pointing and following this gesture with your gaze enables two people to focus on the same object or event and interact with each other. When children point, adults almost invariably engage and communicate with them about whatever they're pointing to. ("Yes, that's a doggy," they might say.) But what if you never learned to point? Some autistic children don't point at all. To request something from inside a closet, some kids will just stand in front of it and wait for help to arrive. Some kids will take your hand and lead you to what they want. Some will squeal and jiggle their bodies as they look at whatever is making their world wonderful, but they might not include another person in this enthusiasm through gesture.

When someone does not point to engage you, they may use other body language. Some people may interact by leaning the weight of their bodies against you. They will get into your space to gain your attention.

I'm a space invader, and sometimes I get in others' personal space. I am also a toucher, a hugger, and a hand-holder. I'll touch a person's arm when they are telling me a story or rub a person's back if they're sad or need encouragement. I express my affection through touch, though I do try to curb my literally touchy-feely ways. That's because I know that being touched is not everyone's cup of tea. My idea of personal space can be very different from someone else's and all of us need to be aware of other people's space boundaries.

In my early years of teaching, I played a social-skills video (yes, I do mean a VHS tape) for a class. The video explained personal space and was demonstrated by two actors.

"When we have a conversation, the rule is to stay one arm's length away from the other person," the narrator stated. One actor lifted his hand and placed his fingertips on the other actor's shoulder. This gesture was repeated several times, both actors taking turns placing their hand on the other's shoulder before beginning a conversation.

I didn't think much of it until I was on playground duty at lunchtime and saw one of the students from the class approach a teacher. He reached his arm up and placed it on the teacher's shoulder, shuffled backward a little so his arm was fully outstretched and straightened, then began to talk. I giggled. I knew what tomorrow's lesson would be. I needed to fill in the gap that the old VHS tape had not: we measure proximity in our minds, not literally with our arms.

Some people struggle with the concept of personal space and may stand too close or too far from others. Some may use hand gestures in unique ways or use almost no gestures at all. Some may have difficulty understanding the gestures of others or may miss visual cues. And some may misinterpret nonverbal communication.

Binh and I were friends. It was an unlikely friendship—I was in my thirties and Binh was ten years younger. I liked to move, and Binh liked to sit still. I liked the outdoors, and Binh liked artificial light. I liked the sun, and Binh hated it. In fact, Binh believed that anyone who liked to sunbathe was not "friendable." According to Binh, if you liked to lie in the sun and get a tan, you were exposing yourself to skin cancer, and therefore you obviously didn't care about living a long life. Binh didn't want friends who were so flippant or had such short-term thinking. After all, he explained, they wouldn't be around for long, and who wants to have a time-limited friend? Luckily for me, I'm freckly and pale and a believer in SPF 50 sunscreen.

Binh and I had met through a committee at the organization where I worked. Binh was the chair of a client committee that drove the organization's strategic direction, and we were often sent to networking events together to increase the visibility of the organization. He was the voice of the clients, and I was his wingman. We were a great team—he was straightforward and spoke with conviction about the needs of people with disabilities, and I was able to back him up with the jargon of government policy and funding. One of the main goals of these events was to build relationships with potential funders, which meant they were all about the schmooze. And Binh hated to schmooze.

Binh was a car fanatic and could give you detailed information about the make and model of your car, its fuel efficiency, and how it compared to similar models. He was also a great advocate for disability rights and could talk your ear off about that topic. But if you wanted to chat about the weather, the weekend's football game, or your child's school trip, Binh would disengage entirely. Like many people, he had difficulty understanding the strange social dance of small talk.

One night Binh and I attended a ball for a disability-inclusion award, and we had been stuck for some time talking with a particularly dry man who worked for a state government department. He made comments on the catering for the event and his recent holiday, but this idle chitchat didn't interest Binh. The civil servant didn't seem to notice, and he continued to speak *at* Binh, telling him some of his outdated thoughts about people with disabilities. Almost as bad, he appeared to have no interest in cars.

We've all been in situations like this that we are desperate to get out of. In this moment, people use their eyes to send a message to a friend, partner, or colleague saying, *Please get me out of this conversation.*

As the public servant droned on, I tried to signal my annoyance to Binh by rolling my eyes in a subtle way. My body was oriented toward him, so the bureaucrat couldn't see my face. It wasn't exaggerated or obvious; it was simply a slight movement of my eyes. I was sending Binh a message saying, *This guy is a nitwit!* But I forgot in that moment that Binh found the subtlety of nonverbal communication complex and difficult. He didn't perceive the message I was trying to convey.

"Jodi!" he exclaimed. "Why are you rolling your eyes? Do you have something in your eye?"

I threw him a glare—*Binnhhhhhhh!*—but it only made it worse.

"Jodi! Are you about to have a seizure?" he blurted out.

I was busted. The public servant, who hadn't picked up on our boredom, definitely knew the meaning of the eye roll. "How rude" was all he said before walking away. We didn't speak to him again for the rest of the night, and I was left wondering how body language could communicate one thing to one person but something completely different to another.

At university when I was learning to be a counselor, I was trained in neurotypical social skills. I was taught to look closely at a person's body language and interpret it. In counseling, you're watching for the match between a person's words, emotion, and body language. You're also looking for the mismatch, when the words spoken and a person's body language convey different meanings. After years of working with autistic people, I have learned that this incongruence is a common feature of autism. And it means that I have thrown my neurotypical-based method of reading body language out the window.

I have learned that a person's slouch may not indicate boredom, that a dramatic story can be told without sweeping arm movements, and that crossed arms and a turned-away body are not necessarily signs that someone does not want to engage. I have learned that I shouldn't expect a neurodivergent person to use neurotypical nonverbal communication because they're not neurotypical. But I have also had to teach many neurodivergent people what neurotypical people *expect* to see and how their body language could be interpreted. I've had to explain that crossing your arms when you're cold might be viewed as defensive and linking your hands behind your head may be seen as cocky and not just as a stretch. We all have difficulty deciphering body language, because the way we gesture and our capacity to read and comprehend each other's bodies is just as diverse as we are.

Dennis and his teacher both needed a translator in nonverbal communication because they were speaking a different language. Because Dennis wasn't nodding, his teacher thought that he wasn't paying attention, and this also meant she wasn't getting the affirmation that she so desperately needed. When I explained to her that she felt snubbed by Dennis because she was missing the subtle movement of the nod, she laughed at herself.

"I didn't realize I needed that level of student feedback!"

Dennis also learned some new tricks. We taught him what his neurotypical teachers might expect to see as the nonverbal cues of engagement and attentiveness. He wasn't asked to change the way he used his body, but he was made aware of how his body language could be perceived. We looked at pictures and videos of different postures and of people sitting up straight, tracking a speaker by moving their heads, and, of course, nodding. "Wow, how do people ever concentrate when they have to think about all of this?" Dennis asked.

I'll tell you a secret: Dennis taught me just how much neurotypical people expect the nod, and I have sometimes used this to my advantage. If I'm attending a social event and I'm talking with someone whose ignorance makes my toes curl, I just stop nodding. It's hard to do, because it's built into my brain, but it's incredible to see how quickly a neurotypical person will cease trying to engage with me when I don't nod. I can see it in their eyes, the confusion. I haven't left—I am still standing right there—but I can see they sense that something is off, and they'll shuffle their shoes, look around the room, and find an excuse to move on. Neurotypical people are often desperate for the nod of approval because it is the unspoken gesture of *Yep, you're all good.*

Our bodies talk, and they talk a lot. We use them to communicate, but we all use them differently. If we just think of neurodivergent body language as being culturally different from neurotypical language, maybe we can view the differences as simply that.

After all, I am not going to use my thumb and forefinger to form an O in Brazil, because that is *not* okay.

# 15

# Joseph's *Mona Lisa*

Sexual harassment and *stalking* were listed as reasons for Joseph's referral to me. He had been expelled from college and there had been police intervention. I had an idea in my head of what Joseph would look like: big, brash, and a little scary. He was the complete opposite: slight and short with baby-smooth skin. During our first appointment, he was aloof, distant, and shy, and he didn't speak first or initiate conversation. If I asked a question, he answered with a short, concise response, but other than that, he just sat in silence, watched, and waited.

There was one topic, however, that Joseph could talk about endlessly: *Game of Thrones*. He had read all the books and watched all the episodes of the TV series too many times to count. He knew the backstory of every character, how the stories interconnected, and the history of each family. He also knew about the "making of" and could tell you every country where the series had been filmed, how many extras had been on the set, the names of the multiple directors (including the only woman, Michelle MacLaren), and how CGI and other technology had been used in individual episodes. Joseph's love of *Game of Thrones* had sparked an interest in filmmaking, so he had enrolled in a media course at his local college.

But something other than film had engaged him: a girl who looked exactly like Daenerys Stormborn of the House Targaryen, First of Her Name, the Unburnt, Queen of the Andals and the First Men, Khaleesi of the Great Grass Sea, Breaker of Chains, and Mother of Dragons.

Joseph had locked eyes with her across a crowded room. Well, he had not actually locked eyes *with* her; Joseph had just locked eyes *on* her. Once he saw her, he was *in*. Joseph followed her every step and watched her every move. He watched her when she arrived at college and got off the bus, he watched her as she walked from class to class, he watched her as she sat in the cafeteria. He watched and stared. And "Daenerys" had become frightened.

In *Game of Thrones*, Daenerys wasn't scared of anything, but this student wasn't leading soldiers into battle for the Iron Throne. For her, Joseph's unblinking gaze was more unnerving than any White Walker, and he just didn't understand why.

The English language is filled with expressions to describe eyes and how people use them: *puppy-dog eyes, having a twinkle in the eye, kind eyes, tired eyes, piercing eyes,* and *shifty eyes*. There's the *dirty look,* the *side-eye,* and *come-to-bed eyes.* Eyes express emotions; we use them to communicate with one another and to connect. We also use them to understand where people's attention is focused, to predict their behavior, and to understand their moods.

Our eyes convey a myriad of emotions through subtle shifts and changes. We perceive the feelings of others through the size of their pupils, how open or closed their eyes are, the distance between their eyes and their eyebrows, and even the slope of the eyebrows. (I have always been so impressed by people who can raise just one eyebrow!) We watch the wrinkles and crinkles around the eyes, nose, and temples, and we understand a person's intention through the movement and direction of their gaze.

Human eyes are unique and distinct from the eyes of all other animals. We're the only mammals with whites that surround the whole eyeball. This allows us to follow each other's gaze. If you are sitting and talking with someone and they shift their eyes to look out a window, you are so attuned to the white that surrounds the iris that you will look out the window too. You want to see what they see. We use our eyes to indicate direction and to request. We use them to agree or disagree, to encourage, and to send messages of boredom. When we interact with others, our eyes will jump and dance and dart or well with tears or appear completely blank and glaze over. The amount of emotion and thought we communicate with our eyes is colossal.

Humans are sensitive to eye contact from others very early in life. Within a few days of birth, a baby will gaze at a face that gazes at them. A baby's eyes are huge relative to the head, so adults are drawn into them and into the wonder of it all. We believe the statements of those who readily make eye contact, and when a person makes eye contact with us, we perceive that they're listening. There is an assumption that people who make eye contact are confident and sincere, that they are sending the message *I am present and with you.*

People can have a whole conversation with just a few glances. Recently my parents came for a visit. My father, who was struggling with pain, had been a little short in his communication and had snapped at my mom. It was a yap that expressed his frustration, not a bite. My mother and I caught each other's eye and, in silence, had a complete conversation. *Wow, that was a bit snappy,* I said by widening my eyes slightly in surprise. *Yes, it was,* she replied, her eyes latching onto mine, then her gaze softened. *But not to worry. We understand why and sometimes you need to let moments like this slide.* I looked at her with deep respect — *You're so good, Mom* — and my mom's eyes crinkled at the edges.

In Western cultures, eye contact is socially appropriate, but in many other cultures, this isn't the case. In fact, it can be a sign of disrespect. For Aboriginal Australians and in some Asian and South American countries, making direct eye contact can be considered rude. This also depends on to whom you are speaking and your relationship with that person.

In fact, how you use your eyes depends on where you live, whom you are with, and what circumstances you are in. We have all been in situations where we avert our eyes to give others privacy. In places in the world where families live together in small rooms, averting the eyes is the only way to give each other space and a sense of dignity.

When my daughter was a teenager, we traveled to Japan and stayed in hotels with shared bathrooms. On the first night, she made me check to see that there was no one else in the bathroom. "Nope, no one there," I stated, and only then would she enter. At fourteen, she was still feeling her way in her new body. For a couple of years prior to this trip, she had been locking her new body behind the doors of our home, but here in Japan, there was nowhere to hide. That first night, her need for privacy was extreme. She had grown up in a culture that made her believe that "everyone" would be looking. In the few weeks we spent in Japan, I watched my daughter learn the power of the eyes. We bathed every day in shared hotel baths and *onsens,* and on one of our final days, we used a *sentō*, a public bath-house, in the city we were visiting.

The changing room there was packed with women of all sizes, shapes, and ages. The eldest were wrinkled and skinny with bent backs and tired bones, the youngest were just toddlers, and there were women of every age in between. My fourteen-year-old Western, Instagram-scrolling daughter walked in, stripped, and wandered fully naked across the room. She had learned that here among many, she could have complete privacy. No one was looking. Everyone was giving each other dignity and respect just by knowing where to direct their eyes.

We learn some of the basic skills of how to use our eyes in childhood. It's not unusual to hear parents encourage their young children to look at people when interacting with them. "Look at Jodi when you say hello," my neighbors say to their child when we greet each other in the yard. Adults are constantly teaching children social skills, but the skills being taught are neurotypical social-interaction skills. Autistic people engage with the world in a different manner, and neurotypical people need to adjust the way they interact to truly embrace this difference.

Many years ago, when I was first teaching and working in the disability sector, the staff constantly used the refrain "Look at me" to get a student to listen. It seems absurd now, but back then we didn't understand why autistic people struggled with eye contact. We also didn't understand that by asking a person to look in our eyes, we were, in fact, interfering with their communication and comprehension.

Many autistic people have explained to me that they cannot do three things at once. "I can look at you and hear the words you say, but then I can't process those words. If I don't look at you, then I am able to really hear what you say and process the words you are saying." This makes sense, doesn't it? Most people don't really need their eyes to listen. Eyes send the speaker a message. When you look at the person talking, you are saying, *I hear you.* But some people who are forced to make eye contact lose their ability to listen.

Nobody makes consistent eye contact. We look at each other and then look away to think about what we are hearing and process the information. Scientists have shown that people tend to look to the right if they are imagining something and to the left if they are remembering. Looking away gives us time to think.

Sometimes the best communication happens when we are not looking at one another. When working with autistic people, I like to think about the communication that takes place between two people when they are fishing, sitting side by side on a park bench looking out at the view, or lying next to each other in bed in the dark. The eyes are not needed in these moments when some of the greatest honesty and truth can be shared.

One young man, Ziggy, came to see me for counseling every two weeks for months and never made eye contact with me. When I first met him, his difficulty with eye contact was evident; he looked everywhere but in my direction. I set up the room so that he was never under pressure to look at me, and I let him know that I didn't expect or need that from him. The common counseling technique of sitting face-to-face was thrown out; Ziggy and I sat side by side, sometimes at a table, where we drew pictures so that we didn't focus on each other, and sometimes on the couch. I never sat across from him because I wanted us to connect, and Ziggy could not connect with me with his eyes.

It's said that our eyes are the windows to our souls, as they display so much emotion. Neurotypical people instinctively read the thoughts and emotions of others through their eyes, but for some autistic people, the constant shift and changes in emotions displayed in the eyes can be complex and difficult to process. "I just can't take on all the thoughts and feelings in someone's eyes" is a consistent explanation I've heard. Some autistic people say eye contact makes them feel uncomfortable, that it's "bewildering" or even "grueling." Simone would give me a fleeting eye gaze maybe once in an hour-long therapy session; Charmaine appeared to be looking at me but in fact looked only at my forehead and lips; and Alec looked at my eyes, but not really. He told me that he was taught to make eye contact, but he found it way too hard, so he came up with a handy strategy: He looked at a person's eyes but did not focus. He kept the eyes in a blur.

Eye contact can be unnerving. We all know what it's like when someone never breaks eye contact; we look away to avoid the intensity of their gaze. Neurotypical people understand that eye contact is important, but they do not maintain it at all times. In fact, they maintain eye contact for only about three seconds before glancing away in most day-to-day interactions. Three seconds is just about perfect, but nine seconds is considered intimidating.

Lack of eye contact is one component of an autism diagnosis but it's only a small piece of a bigger story. Level of shyness, a person's self-esteem, hypersensitivity, cultural identity, and gender can also affect how people use their eyes. By understanding that none of us locks pupil to pupil for extended periods, maybe we can shift the focus away from eye contact as necessary and think about how we can connect in different ways.

* * *

In Joseph's case, the way he used his eyes not only created difficulty in his interpersonal connections but also gave him a reputation on campus as a creep. Although I would never ask an autistic person (or anyone) to make eye contact with me, Joseph needed support in understanding that how he used his eyes had an impact on others.

"Three seconds, Joseph," I explained. "We look at someone for about three seconds, and then we look away."

"Then why do they put chairs in art galleries?" he asked.

I was perplexed. What did art galleries have to do with any of this?

"In art galleries," he explained, "they put chairs in front of the paintings that people love most. When you really love something, you want to look. When you think everything about them is glorious, you want to keep looking and don't want to stop. In an art gallery there are chairs so you can do this. You wouldn't turn away from the *Mona Lisa*, would you?"

And once again, my mind was blown by the diversity of how people see and perceive the world.

So I shared with Joseph the Mills & Boon technique. Mills & Boon publishes sappy romance novels, and in my early teenage years, I'd raid my grandmother's bookshelf for them. (Unfortunately, Gran stopped buying these books when she felt the protagonists were starting to have sexual encounters too quickly.) I devoured these stories and thought that Mills & Boon would give me all the answers to how to get a prince or princess to arrive on my doorstep on that white stallion. The books follow a romance formula, and nearly every one has a specific scene where the star-crossed lovers meet for the first time.

*Their eyes locked across a crowded room.* We all know this scene. You've seen it in movies and may even have experienced it yourself. It's that moment when your eyes meet, you hold each other's gaze, and this gaze is extended for just a micro-millisecond. Something passes between you. But that moment of locking eyes is *not* the important one. It is what happens next: *And then they turned away.*

The moment we look away is key. In this moment, our hearts flutter and we hope that what we expressed with our eyes and what we perceived is true. We break eye contact and turn away—and then we turn and look again. We look back over our shoulders in the hope that they'll be looking back too, that our hope will be reciprocated.

Some people believe in love at first sight, but it's actually the breaking of eye contact and then the returned second glance that makes it real.

# 16

# Frankie's Magic Carpet

Frankie looked like a four-year-old Snow White, all porcelain skin and jet-black hair — but bluebirds did not land on her hand, because she was the opposite of a gentle and demure singing princess. Frankie moved through the world in a rough-and-tumble way, always on the go, somersaulting and twirling and hanging upside down to see the land inverted. She was hard to keep up with; she darted from one activity to another, leaving traces of her existence in scattered pencils, abandoned blocks, and discarded puzzle pieces.

Frankie was a whirlwind of a child, sweeping up objects and then strewing them in her wake. She could never sit still. Except when she was watching a Disney movie.

Frankie loved Disney movies and would watch them over and over. Like any child who wants to have the same books read to them on repeat, Frankie would get on a roll with a particular movie and be stuck on it for months before jumping to a new one and starting the cycle again. *The Lion King* had a great run, and both *101 Dalmatians* and *102 Dalmatians* had once been in high rotation. She loved the old classics, like *Dumbo*, *The Jungle Book*, and *Robin Hood*, and as a result her home was full of elephants, bears, and singing foxes, all blaring nonstop from the TV.

Frankie constantly repeated phrases from her current favorite movie under her breath. They were a persistent mantra in her waking hours, whispered not quite loud enough for others to understand what she was saying. Frankie didn't converse in the same way that many other children do. Apart from repeating lines from movies, she had limited speech for communicating with others. She'd take your hand to show you what she wanted— for instance, she'd lead you to the back door so you could let her outside. And she could say a few things, like *milk* and *cookie*, which were her particular favorites. But aside from that, her inter-action with others was nearly always based on Disney quotes.

She was a walking Disney movie, and because Frankie's family wanted to engage with her, they immersed themselves in the world of Disney too. When Frankie became obsessed with *The Little Mermaid*, her family watched the movie with her hundreds of times. They could sing along to "Under the Sea" and "Kiss the Girl." They knew Ariel's collection of gadgets and gizmos, whosits and whatsits and thingamabobs. They knew Ariel delighted in combing her hair with a fork and that Ursula the sea witch was a crazy combination of human and octopus. They knew the movie by heart, so when Frankie quoted lines from the film, they could answer with the next line.

" 'This, I haven't seen this in years. This is wonderful,' " Frankie would coo.

" 'What is it?' " her family would ask.

" 'A banded, bulbous snarfblatt!' "

A few weeks after I met Frankie, she moved from *The Little Mermaid* to *Aladdin*, and hearing the words of Robin Wil-liams's robust Genie emerging from her little mouth brought about many giggles.

One day, I visited Frankie at the childcare center she attended three days a week. I was there to help create a routine for her so that she could be more engaged in the activities of the day. During outdoor play, Frankie took hold of my hand and led me to the swings. I knew she was giving me a *Jodi, push me!* physical prompt. (All kids know swinging is better with a push.) As I stood behind Frankie and pushed her with the rhythm of physics, Frankie found a way to show me her appreciation.

" 'I'm getting kinda fond of you, kid,' " she parroted in her Genie voice. " 'Not that I wanna pick out curtains or anything.' "

I couldn't have been happier in that moment. Frankie was communicating with me in her way. She was expressing her thoughts and feelings through the language of *Aladdin*. She did not have the words for *I'm happy* or *I like you* or even *Thank you*, but she did have the Genie.

And the Genie could express himself very well.

It takes incredible skill to memorize large amounts of dialogue, but most of us have the capacity to remember and repeat at least a smidgen of what we hear. Some people can quote lines from their favorite films at exactly the right time in exactly the right way. These moments can make people around them laugh or roll their eyes, but if those people know the movie too, it helps them connect.

My brother could quote every line from *Trading Places* as a kid and took particular pleasure in putting on Eddie Murphy's multiple voices. I have a friend who throws out lines from *Shrek* as if they were meant to be in everyday conversation. (And she is usually right: "After a while you learn to ignore the names people call you and just trust who you are.") Another friend is a compulsive quoter from films as diverse as *Full Metal Jacket* and *Zoolander*.

Most of us have quotes like these stored in our brains, lines from movies we have watched and lyrics from songs we have heard. These lines echo in our minds, but sometimes the words or lyrics become caught and we repeat them over and over. We hear a snippet of a song on our way to work and then those same few bars and words repeat in our minds all day long. Psychologists call this "involuntary musical imagery," but most of us know it as an earworm.

An earworm is usually a tiny fragment of a song, maybe two or three bars of music and lyrics, that your memory gets stuck on, the same line again and again, and that worm can drive you to despair until it leaves your head. Music is defined by repetition, and it is incredible — and sometimes annoying — that we can retain the melody, beats, and lyrics of so many songs and tunes.

Echolalia, or echoing what you hear, is a beautiful stage in speech and language development. Tiny babies begin to work out how to speak by mimicking the sounds and words and speech patterns of those around them; as adults, we encourage this instinct by using echolalia to teach children to interact with us. We turn our words into the words that *we* want *them* to say. We say "please" and "thank you" when handing toddlers objects to encourage them to do the same, and we coax babies to utter "Mama" and "Dada." Just the other day I watched a woman with two very young children at the market say in the direction of her daughter, "Oh, thank you, Daddy. I love croissants." This mother was speaking the words that she wanted her child to echo. (And I wanted to tell her what a great parent I thought she was.)

We also teach speech and language by using echolalia in more subtle and unconscious ways. For instance, you might call your partner Mom or Dad in front of your children or call your own parents Grandma and Granddad so that the child copies you and calls them by the right relationship name.

Before they learn reciprocal (back-and-forth) language and communication, most children use echolalia to play with words in the early stages of their speech development. Children between eighteen and thirty months will imitate the words and phrases that they hear, but once their language develops and they find their own voices, the adults' voices fade and they speak for themselves. As toddlers become more spontaneous and creative with their speech, they move away from echoed scripts.

Because early communication and social development is based on mimicking, it's natural for kids to parrot language. But when it comes to neurodivergent children, some learn language in their own way.

When Theo was four years old, everyone believed him to be nonspeaking. Theo had an angel's face and big brown eyes with eyelashes that people today would pay hundreds of dollars for. He was a country boy who lived on a farm with his parents and sister, as well as chickens and ducks and cattle dogs. Theo loved the animals, and the animals loved Theo.

Theo hadn't gone through the neurotypical language stages from babbling to using single words to using multiple words. In fact, he just didn't speak at all—or so everyone thought. One day his parents were in the kitchen and heard someone singing, so they went to investigate. Theo, the boy who had never spoken a word, was singing all the words to the nursery rhyme "Itsy Bitsy Spider" in a squeaky but clear voice. His parents were overjoyed. Their boy was *singing!* His father was so excited that he recorded the moment on his phone, just like all proud parents when their children say their first words.

It turns out that while Theo didn't repeat single words or

phrases his parents said in the moment, he could repeat long strings of words he had heard before. He might have heard that nursery rhyme repeatedly at childcare, on TV, or when his sister sang it. He collected these words, repeating them in his mind, and when he was ready, he just sang the lot.

We will never know what triggered this first song, these first spoken words. Perhaps there'd been a spider on the wall in Theo's bedroom. Or maybe it was the rain that came down. Or maybe he'd heard someone say something about sunshine or waterspouts. But for Theo, the words of the nursery rhyme were connected, so once one word was uttered, all the words that followed were spoken too.

Repetition is key in learning language. For some autistic people, watching characters chattering away on a screen provides this consistency, and many kids learn their first words not from their caregivers but from the shows that most entertain them. Learning to speak via television and movies instead of in real-life conversations can have some fascinating results. Over the years, I have been asked why some autistic people speak in accents. In Australia, some autistic adults have American or British accents despite never having visited these countries; I have spent time with autistic children who speak with a Latino accent like Dora the Explorer or with a British accent like Thomas the Tank Engine. Even though their families speak to them in Aussie accents, they learn language from TV shows and movies, mimicking accents from around the world.

One advantage to learning language from movies is that a film you've seen a dozen times is predictable and reliable, unlike a person. People—well, we can be very inconsistent in the way we communicate! We might say things differently or use the same words but not mean the same thing. But song lyrics and lines spoken in movies *do* remain consistent. C will always follow B in the ABC song; Romeo and Juliet will not miraculously live happily ever after; and Queen's "Bohemian Rhapsody" will always be one of the best earworms ever. (Sorry—now that'll be stuck in your head too.) We have to thank the screenwriters and lyricists for making the language of film and music so meaningful to so many of us.

There was one language the Genie didn't speak that Frankie *needed* to learn, a physical one. Swimming.

Frankie lived near the ocean, which meant her brothers and sisters were in the water all day long. Because the family surfed and swam, it was important for Frankie to be safe around water. Her family enrolled her in swimming lessons, but they proved problematic, as she was not able to follow the instructions of the swimming coach. Her parents moved her from group sessions to individual lessons, but that didn't help. Every week the lesson ended in tears—not just Frankie's but also her mom's and the swimming instructor's. No matter how much coaxing and cajoling they did, Frankie would not get in the water. She would sit by the side of the pool and dangle her feet in but would go no farther.

The teacher tried encouraging her by putting toys in the water, but Frankie was not in the least bit interested. Her mom got in the water to show Frankie how great it was, but Frankie just walked away.

"Jump in, Frankie!" her mom called. "Come on in, Frankie!" the teacher added. "It's fun!"

Frankie was having none of it.

They were not speaking Frankie's language.

I have done some strange things in my life to try to connect with autistic people. And I knew that if I wanted to connect with Frankie, I needed to learn the language of *Aladdin*. So I watched it over and over. I learned all the lines and what those lines represented and worked out how to use them in the perfect moments. Armed with this new language, I went to Frankie's swimming lessons to be her translator.

Frankie sat on the side of the pool. Her mother and swimming teacher had been trying to coax her in, but as usual, she wouldn't budge.

I slipped into the pool so that the water was up to my chest. I stood in front of Frankie and began speaking to her in Aladdinish.

"'You don't want to go for a ride, do you?'" I said, imagining myself on Aladdin's magic carpet, hovering below Frankie's balcony. "'We could get out of the palace. See the world.'"

Frankie looked up at the ceiling. She took a breath and recited the next line, the line she knew so well. "'Is it safe?'" Frankie replied with Jasmine's words, turning to look out over the water.

"'Sure, do you trust me?'" I stretched out my hand to her.

"'What?'"

"'Do you trust me?'"

And seeing my hand outstretched, reaching for hers, Frankie stepped off the balcony and into the pool.

# 17

# Leo's Madonna

Leo and I have been friends for more than thirty years. We live far apart but see each other whenever we are in the same town. Leo and I met when I was employed as his support worker in my twenties. While I might have helped Leo work out the math when shopping, showed him how to read the sides of the packets so he could follow the cooking directions, and taught him how to travel by bus, he helped me by filling me with laughter. After I left that position, we formed a true friendship.

Leo was in his late teens when we started hanging out together. The best and only way I can describe him is that he was a complete goof. He talked nonstop about the things he loved — mostly bad TV sitcoms and the most attractive characters on them. He always wore his favorite football jersey, and when heading out, he would connect his keys to his belt loop with a chain and tuck them into his pocket.

Leo had no control over the volume of his voice. He'd think he was speaking in an indoor voice but the person he was speaking to would ask him why he was shouting. Leo was loud at home, loud in the library, and loud in stores. His voice boomed. When he went out for dinner, every person in the restaurant knew he felt that pineapple had no place on pizza.

Luckily, Leo loved the outdoors. He had a job with a disability-employment company doing garden maintenance, and a pumpkin he'd grown had won an award at the local horticultural show. He loved to fish and he'd taught me how to bait a hook, cast a rod, and gut what we caught.

But most of all, Leo loooovvved Madonna.

Leo had Madonna cassettes (we weren't cool enough for CDs yet) that he played on repeat. He would sing "Like a Virgin" and "Like a Prayer" and break out into "Vogue" dance moves. He wore Madonna T-shirts and had Madonna posters on his bedroom walls. He even had a photo of Madonna, cut from a magazine, in his wallet. He had a massive crush on Madonna.

In 1993, the movie *Body of Evidence*, starring Leo's all-time-favorite person, hit the cinemas. He talked about it constantly before its release date, and I promised to take him the very first day it opened at our local movie theater. *Body of Evidence* was about a court case in which Madonna's character needed defending, and Willem Dafoe's character was defending her. That's what I thought, anyway—a good courtroom drama, and Leo would be delighted to see Madonna on the screen even if he didn't understand all of the legal jargon.

I should have read a little more about this movie. I should have noticed that Madonna was naked on one movie poster and that she and Willem Dafoe were locked in a passionate embrace on another. Maybe the fact that it was rated R should have clued me in, but Leo and I were both over eighteen, so I just went to the movies with Leo.

What happened next changed how I and everyone else in

that cinema viewed Madonna forever. But while my thoughts were quietly whispered to Leo, Leo's were projected through the auditorium via his built-in megaphone.

I have always hated my voice. We all have weird self-esteem issues, and for me it is my broad accent. For a long time, I believed I didn't sound like an intelligent person, and I wanted to sound smart.

I have a friend who is a speech pathologist, and I used to ask her if she could Eliza Doolittle me. My friend, who is years younger than I am, had not been exposed to the 1964 film *My Fair Lady* and had no idea what I was talking about. I gave her a DVD of the musical, which is about a poor Cockney flower seller who is groomed to be presented as a high-society lady. I wanted to be able to say "The rain in Spain stays mainly in the plain" in an equally refined manner. I hoped that she would take on the role of Professor Higgins and help me learn to speak with a plum in my mouth.

"No," she said. "I love your voice!"

Some people have more distinctive voices than others, voices that are immediately recognizable, and most people can identify specific singers, actors, and sports commentators based on their voices alone. But all voices are like fingerprints; each one has its own individual sound. Even though many voices are similar, they all have their own distinguishing features.

The human voice is not just about the words; voice also conveys *meaning*. The vocal and intonation tools we use to enhance what we say—pitch, tone, speed, volume, and inflection, the study of which is called prosody—amplify the words we speak and sometimes even change what the words mean.

Try saying this out loud:

*Really* (meaning "I don't quite believe you")
*Really* (meaning "I am telling the truth")

Even the slightest difference in intonation can change a word's meaning.

When you're excited or anxious, the muscles in your vocal cords tense, and your pitch rises. When you're relaxed, your pitch is lower. Tone is the pattern of highs and lows in pitch, and inflection is using pitch in a word or a sentence. (In Australia we often raise the pitch at the end of a sentence, which makes everything sound like a question.) In addition to pitch, adjusting speed and tempo changes the meaning of words. And then there are accents, clarity, pronunciation, and projection. Voices are simple, aren't they? (Said with sarcasm.)

Irene had no rise or fall in her speech. She spoke in a monotone but her words were far from monotonous. The stories Irene told me in counseling were jaw-dropping. They often involved the escapades of a young woman in her early twenties and lots of "drugs, sex, and rock and roll." Irene's eyeliner was thick and smudged; she always looked like she had just woken up after a big night out and hadn't removed her makeup. She loved safety pins and used them to hold together the rips in her jeans and wore them in chains as earrings. Her shirts and bag were covered in buttons with slogans like GIRL POWER and WELL-BEHAVED WOMEN RARELY MAKE HISTORY. She was brilliant, but she sounded like a professor I once had who could put the class to sleep with just his voice.

She and I had to navigate this in the way we communicated.

"Wow, this is an exciting activity," she said as we created a list of what a respectful relationship should entail.

"Oh, that's good," I replied.

"Jodi, I was being sarcastic!"

But how was I to know? Sarcasm is complex. You know someone is being sarcastic by detecting the subtleties in the tone of voice, the pauses around the words, and where the stress is placed. Some autistic people cannot detect the inflection and tone that create sarcasm, and some people (neurodivergent or otherwise) don't employ the subtle pause needed to relay that they're being ironic. Sarcasm, irony, and jokes all need these slight shifts and changes. If you don't or can't register them, the joke falls flat.

The way we project our words adds to the message we want to convey. We increase and decrease volume to reflect the environment we are in, our proximity to others, and the intensity of our emotions. We'll speak louder to make an impact and whisper to express vulnerability.

For many people, working out the right decibel level to speak at can be out of their conscious control. People often say to me, "I heard you before I saw you," because I'm loud. *Overly enthusiastic* is how I like to describe it, but I do try to tone it down and speak with a quieter voice because I understand that not everyone needs to know what a great day I'm having.

My daughter, like the majority of children, had to learn the art of the inside voice. When she was young, we lived in Singapore, an island with a blend of races, cultures, and ethnicities. One day while we were on a train, she spotted a Sikh man sitting across from us.

"Mom, why does that man have a scarf around his head?" she asked in a voice that echoed through the quiet carriage.

I was embarrassed, and the man caught my eye. What was I to do? It was an innocent question, asked with great curiosity. I went to hush her, but this lovely man answered in a voice just as loud as hers.

"This is called a turban," he said, smiling at her.

Children ask these questions before they learn to adjust their volume and before they understand social etiquette. We learn through social trial and error when the questions inside our heads can be spoken and when they need to stay in our thoughts. We learn when we should speak quietly into another's ear with a cupped hand and when we can scream that same sentiment from the rooftops. I'm still learning when to turn the volume down! Just today I apologized to a café full of people after I had announced way too loudly to my friend that I had sand in my pants.

Some autistic people may have difficulties regulating their volume throughout their lives. They may have trouble sensing their own volume or struggle to filter out background noise and feel they need to talk over it. Some may not be aware of what conversations or questions should be kept private, and some may not realize that not every thought needs to be spoken out loud.

We are constantly imparting meaning through our tone, volume, pitch, and speed. But we don't all speak in the same way, and we need to cut each other some slack. Not all of us are master communicators; at best, we are lifetime apprentices.

Leo and I settled into the cinema for the matinee with giant boxes of popcorn and humongous Cokes. As the multiple ads told us what was coming soon, I relaxed in my seat and put my feet up on the chair in front of me. (We could still do that in those days.)

And then the movie began.

Within the first three minutes, Madonna was naked and having sex. And the sex scenes kept on coming. It was the 1993 version of *Fifty Shades of Grey*. There were belts and dripping wax. There was champagne being licked from chests and breasts and torsos. I cringed and sweated and looked sideways at Leo, whose eyes were as big as saucers.

*Oh no,* I thought, *what have we gotten ourselves into?*

But then came the garage scene.

Madonna's character enters a darkly lit, multistory garage and climbs onto the hood of a stranger's car. She slips her skirt up to her hips and stands there waiting as Willem Dafoe approaches her. With his face at Madonna's waist, he slowly removes her underwear, and she, with the strength of someone who has been performing chin-ups at the gym her entire life, raises her hands to the rafters, hoists herself up, and wraps her legs around Dafoe's head.

It was intense and filled with lust and want. And then...

"Jodi, what is Madonna doing?" Leo asked, loud enough for the whole cinema to hear.

I sank into my seat as the people around us giggled.

"I'll tell you later," I whispered to him from the side of my mouth.

"But, Jode," Leo trumpeted again with gusto, "why does Madonna have her legs wrapped around his head? Is she trying to do a wrestling hold on him? Is she trying to strangle him?"

And during a scene when the audience should have been feeling the racing of their own hearts and pondering their own upper-body strength, the entire cinema exploded in laughter.

# 18

# Nash's Sneakers

Nash arrived at the office with a new pair of shoes still in their shoebox. This was bizarre, because Nash was not a shopper.

Nash had worn the same clothes for the past two years. Even on the hottest of summer days, Nash wore his one pair of baggy jeans and one of his three T-shirts, featuring Chewbacca, Yoda, or Jabba the Hutt. These clothes lasted a long time because Nash never washed them. After each session I had to open my office windows and air out the room.

At twenty-five, Nash had no awareness of his own personal hygiene or his pungent smell. Once I felt I'd gotten to know him, I mentioned daily showering, using soap, and why deodorant was a handy thing.

It had taken me a few weeks to feel that our relationship was solid enough that I could bring up the delicate subject of "Nash, you smell," but from the day we met, Nash always spoke his mind. He immediately let me know his opinions on everything:

"Jodi, your breath smells of coffee."

"Jodi, that dress is terrible."

"Jodi, your hair up like that makes you look old."

Nash had no filter and said exactly what he thought, so he assumed that everyone else did the same.

"Wow, Nash—new shoes!" I exclaimed. "I'm surprised."

"The guy in the shop said, 'You should buy them.'"

"Did he say 'You should buy them' as an encouragement or as a suggestion?"

"He just said, 'You should buy them.' So I did."

It takes a lot of effort for people to comprehend one another. We use a lot of words to try to communicate—the average English-speaking adult has a vocabulary of between 20,000 and 35,000 words—but not all of them are as straightforward as they seem. English is a particularly weird language: Why do we have so many words that sound the same but have different meanings? Why do we have *prey* and *pray* and *blew* and *blue*, *sell* and *cell*, and *by*, *buy*, and *bye*?

Words can be confusing but also beautiful, and the way we string them together can bring them to life and make them vivid. Language can be playful; we can make meaning from mental images. In German, *Sein Herz auf der Zunge tragen* translates to "Carry one's heart on the tongue"—it means to be open with your emotions. In French, *Occupe-toi de tes oignons* translates to "Take care of your own onions," but what it really means is "Mind your own business." And in Indonesian, *Makan angin* translates to "Eat wind" but actually means to relax or take a vacation.

I love metaphors and use a lot of them; it gives language color. People use them so much that they may not even know they're doing it. But not everyone understands metaphors.

Many of my autistic clients have taught me just how often I drop metaphors into my day-to-day conversations. Sri was one of these people.

Me: Hey, Sri, can I pick your brain?
Sri: Absolutely not, that is disgusting.
Me: The world is your oyster.
Sri: I don't like oysters.
Me: So, if you have your ducks in a row —
Sri: I don't live on a farm. I don't have any ducks.

Sri taught me to laugh at my own words. She took whatever came out of my mouth as meaning exactly what it sounded like. One day we had a cup of tea and some chocolate together. I put my wrapper inside the cup when I had finished, and Sri did the same. Then, wanting to be helpful, she picked up our cups to take them to the sink.

"Just throw them in the trash," I said.

After she left, I went to wash the cups and couldn't find them. Sri had thrown the chocolate wrappers, cups, and spoons in the bin! Something had gotten lost in translation.

Language can be literal—the words mean exactly what they seem to mean. Or it can be figurative—the words mean something other than their literal definitions. Literal thinkers like Sri hear words and think of them in concrete terms; they don't see the pictures others are trying to paint with figurative language. Because of this, some autistic people have difficulty understanding phrases when they're flowery and not straightforward and clear.

Many people take for granted that others will comprehend their words, but there can be a breakdown in communication if the intention behind the words is not understood.

I once worked for an organization that helped families understand their children's autism in early childhood. No two families are the same, so this support was always based on an individual family's needs. It was during this time that I learned that the information given to caregivers at the point of diagnosis is not always fully understood.

Clarisa and Ned both had an intellectual disability, and welfare services had requested that we visit to provide guidance on their parenting skills. Max, their four-year-old, had autism, and his eighteen-month-old sister, Nellie, was behind in all of her developmental milestones. A speech pathologist and I visited their home to see what we could do to help.

Before I entered the house, I saw a large tin of cigarette butts outside the front door. It was a huge gallon-size pineapple juice can that overflowed with hundreds and hundreds of butts. It was a sign that no one was smoking inside the house; Clarisa and Ned obviously cared about the health of their children.

It's hard to open your home to a revolving door of welfare workers assessing your needs and those of your children. You'd think that we would have been greeted with disdain, but Ned flung the door open with a wide grin.

"We can use all the help we can get!" he cheerfully announced.

By most people's standards, the house was in disarray. There was stuff everywhere, and by *stuff*, I mean flotsam and jetsam discarded immediately after use. There were dirty clothes and toys and broken bits of household bric-a-brac strewn across every surface. There were used bowls and plates, mugs and cutlery dropped where they had last touched a mouth, still with leftover food caked on the edges. There was, however, a perfectly organized pile in one corner—of pizza boxes.

"Here, take a seat," said Ned as he pushed aside a mound of clothing on the couch. The house smelled of mildew, and the carpet was soggy and spongy underfoot. We sat on a forest of cat hair, surrounded by the mayhem of this family's everyday life.

Coffee was offered. Though some therapists will not accept a drink in a client's home, I'm of the belief that hospitality and generosity are key to relationships, and in some cultures, food means connection. So I accepted. It wasn't the best coffee I had ever tasted, so I sipped it slowly. I knew this was a gesture of welcoming, and their kindness was appreciated, even if their coffeemaking skills weren't.

We heard Max before we saw him. He kept up a running commentary to himself as he bounded down the hall toward us, and he entered the living room like a tumbling circus performer and ricocheted off all the solid surfaces. He might one day be a parkour champion. But not then! Watching him, I was surprised that he had any energy at all.

Max looked like a ghost. His skin was almost translucent, and under his eyes were the dark circles of allergic shiners. He was a stick figure with spindly legs and arms and a round, solid, bloated little tummy. Max was clearly not well, and his parents had taken him to see the doctor.

"The doctor said Max needed to eat spinach to be healthy," Clarisa told us. "We gave it to him, but he just wouldn't eat it."

"So we said to him, 'If you don't eat it now, you get it for breakfast!'" said Ned, finishing where Clarisa left off. "Four days! Four days he wouldn't eat it."

"Did he eat anything else? Did he eat at all?" I asked.

"No, nothing, 'cause we only gave him the spinach."

Clarisa and Ned explained that the doctor had told them Max had to eat steak and spinach, and as they couldn't afford steak, they'd stocked up on frozen spinach. This was microwaved and given to Max at each and every meal. They were trying so hard to be good parents, and following the doctor's orders was good parenting, wasn't it?

"The doctor said that Max needs that thing...what's it called, Ned?" Clarisa asked.

"Iron. Remember, we laughed 'cause we don't even have an iron." Ned chuckled.

Ned and Clarisa had taken the doctor's suggestion literally and didn't understand that Max could eat other iron-rich foods too. Together, we added ground beef, eggs, and peanut butter to his meals, as well as Max's new favorite, spinach and cheese muffins.

Sometimes we need a bit of help to comprehend complex information. Most people expect others to read between the lines of what they're saying and understand the subtext, but this doesn't always happen. I have learned this the hard way.

While studying to become a special-education teacher, I worked in community support with people with disabilities. At the time, I thought I was an exceptional support worker because I was learning strategies and techniques at university and putting these into practice in my job. I was young, and with youth comes a healthy dose of ego. I assumed I was an expert at support work, but Tony taught me otherwise.

Tony was one of four boys. He and his older brother were both autistic, though Tony had an intellectual disability while his brother did not. The other two brothers were neurotypical. Tony was fifteen and learning to be more independent. We would meet after school a couple of times a week. Poor Tony became my practice subject for everything I was learning about developmental disability and autism at university.

Tony and I went to the public swimming pool on our afternoons together. Tony needed help dressing, but he had been practicing how to put on his clothes at home as well as with me after swimming. These were the days before wheelchair-accessible toilets and changing rooms, and for many months Tony had to come into the women's changing rooms with me. Can you imagine that? He was fifteen and had to change in the presence of women and girls. I would take him into a cubicle, but I never felt right about it. For him, having to come into this space took away his dignity, and I had to field many irate comments as to why a teenage boy was in the women's changing room.

Learning to dress yourself is hard. There are many parts of the body that need to be maneuvered to get legs in pants and arms in sleeves. You have to work out whether a shirt is inside out or back to front and manipulate buttons and zippers. It took a long time for Tony to master the art of dressing, and once he had, he wanted to have a go on his own in the men's changing room.

The next time we went swimming, I confidently followed the strategies I had learned at university: (1) analyze the task; (2) break the task into steps; (3) communicate in simple language the sequence of steps to be followed; and (4) check for understanding, comprehension, and retention.

"Okay, Tony," I said. "Go to the changing room. Take off your swimsuit. Have a shower. Get dressed. Meet me back here. Now, can you tell me what you're going to do?"

And Tony repeated it: "Go to the changing room. Take off my swimsuit. Have a shower. Get dressed and come back."

"Okay, let's go," I said.

I thought I'd nailed it! Standing in the shower in the women's changing room, I congratulated myself. *Wow, Jodi Rodgers—you are brilliant at this*, I thought. While I dressed, I went through other tasks in my mind, breaking them down into small steps. How do we brush our teeth, wash our hands, boil a kettle?

And as I was giving myself the Nobel Prize in task analysis, I walked out of the changing room and around the corner and saw Tony standing in the place we'd arranged to meet. His hair was dripping wet and his clothes, although all on in the right direction, were drenched and stuck to his skin. He was a walking waterfall. And he was as pleased as punch with himself.

"I did it, Jodi!" he said, clearly proud. "I went to the changing room, I took off my swimsuit, had a shower, got dressed, and came back here. I did it!"

"But Tony!" I said. "You didn't dry yourself!"

And he looked at me like I was out of my mind. "It wasn't on the list," he replied.

I have remembered this moment hundreds of times during my career. I remember it each and every time things go a little sideways. When things don't quite go according to plan, it's usually because of something I have done—the way I communicated, the way I explained, the way I provided information. I then have to take a look at myself and rethink.

The Nobel Prize remains out of reach thirty years on, and I have never referred to myself as an expert at anything ever again.

Miscommunication happens all the time. It's the confusion between what's been spoken, what was meant, and how it was understood that gets people into hot water. (Another potentially confusing metaphor!) We're not always going to hit the nail on the head, but being a good communicator is not about getting it right every time; it's about attempting to mend the communication breakdowns. Most important, it's about being able to say, "I'm sorry, that's not what I meant," "I'm sorry, that's not what I heard," and "I'm sorry, let's try that again."

\* \* \*

"I don't even want these shoes," Nash said. "I don't even like them."

"It's okay, Nash," I said. "You can always take them back. Don't beat yourself up about it."

"I'd never do that!" he asserted. "Why would I ever bash myself?"

Nash and I spoke a lot that day about his confusion. We spoke about the differing meanings behind the shop assistant's statement. Was it a suggestion that he should buy the shoes? A demand?

"Why didn't he say, 'Are you going to buy those shoes?'" Nash asked. "Because then I would have just said no."

Nash wanted to know why people spoke in riddles. He wanted to know why words had to be a guessing game, why people didn't just cut to the chase. It's no wonder we all get our wires crossed! (Nash, of course, used none of these expressions.)

As our appointment drew to a close, I gathered his file and papers together and stood to indicate our time was up. Nash stood too.

"People are complex, Nash, and sometimes it's really hard to understand each other. Just so you know, I'm here to support you," I said. "I'm not going anywhere."

"Oh, then why are you standing?" replied Nash as he sat back down.

# 19

# Jimmy's Atlas

The kids in Jimmy's class laughed at him. Jimmy was out of sync with the rest of the fourteen-year-olds, and they all knew it.

Before the early 1990s, a diagnosis of autism had to include intellectual disability. In the mainstream schools where I taught, I now know that statistically there must have been autistic kids in every classroom, but at that time, we didn't have a name for it. And because teachers didn't know what the behavioral differences they were observing truly were, autistic students like Jimmy were not getting the support that they needed.

Jimmy was the kid who would be doing the Nutbush dance while everyone else was doing the YMCA. He appeared to have little interest in the social norms of his school environment. While most of the students were conforming to those around them and not wanting to stand out, Jimmy didn't sport the spiky, frosted-tip hairstyle of the rest of the boys; his long hair, which he never wanted to cut, made him distinct and recognizable. While Jimmy's differences were noted by his classmates, he was the type of student who easily flew under the radar of the staff. He was not a young person who demanded attention;

he was quiet, studious, and always completed his homework on time.

One day in geography class, I was asking the students questions and calling on them by name to answer. (If I knew then what I know now, I would not have been calling kids out like that and raising their anxiety.) I asked Jimmy a question just as I had asked the other students, and I expected an immediate response: "Jimmy, what is the capital city of France?"

No response. It was as if he hadn't heard me. A slight lift of the head; nothing else.

*Oh, Jimmy,* I remember thinking. *What am I going to do with you? What will I put down for class participation in your report if you don't participate?*

So I moved on to someone else.

"Beau, what is the capital of Iceland?"

"Hazel, what is the capital of Vietnam?"

Both kids raised their heads, looked straight at me, and quickly answered. And just as I was about to move on to another student...

"Paris!" The word was spoken loudly and with deliberation by Jimmy from his seat in the back of the class. The kids laughed, of course. They all thought that Jimmy was being funny. They thought he was knowingly being disruptive, answering a question a good three minutes after he had been asked.

I thought this too. Initially, I figured that Jimmy had taken up the role of class clown, but I could tell that he was listening because he always gave the correct answer. He just needed more time than the other kids to respond.

This left me wondering: Wasn't it my job to help Jimmy? Wasn't it my job to consider multiple learning styles? After all, teachers are just actors standing in front of a class with a captive audience. Maybe I needed to play a new role just for Jimmy.

It's complex and difficult, this auditory stuff. A word is just a minute sound, and this sound and all the sounds that surround it must be held together while they travel along the neurological pathways in the brain. Once they reach their destination, their meaning must be decoded. We hear the sounds, understand these sounds as words, translate them into meaning, and then form our own sounds into words and have them come out of our mouths. It is really quite amazing that our brains have the capacity to do this—and in microseconds.

Have you ever learned a second language? Learning to communicate in a new language is hard. Can you imagine trying to learn a new language and having someone say, "Will you just hurry up! What is taking you so long? Why aren't you answering me?" The pressure to respond and the anxiety of whether you can do it quickly enough would probably make you give up trying to communicate in that unfamiliar tongue. You would be shy and embarrassed and feel like you were just not smart enough.

I'm a talker and I fill the world with words, but I have learned (through lots of trial and error) that pausing and silences are just as important, if not more important, than words. When you pause, you give others the opportunity to think. A pause after a question or a comment allows people to gather their thoughts before responding. If you do not give people time to process, you might as well be talking to yourself.

When smartphones first came into being, my daughter loved to make voice recordings. She once recorded a conversation we had in her bedroom. When I listened to it, I was shocked. It was not a conversation; it was a monologue.

It started innocently enough: "Can you clean your room?" When she didn't respond, I began issuing multiple instructions: "Clothes off the floor, things into baskets, cups to be taken to the kitchen." Then it built to a crescendo: "If you don't do it now, there is no time...busy week...no laundry can be done...won't have time to dry...cost of using the dryer... impact of dryers on the environment...how will your dance clothes be clean for Saturday...what will your dance teacher say..."

I was on a rant, and I spoke without stopping for breath between my demands, instructions, and rambling thoughts of the future. I heard my daughter's voice only once. "Mom. Slow down."

And she was right. I was not allowing her time to process the one simple instruction that needed to be processed: "Can you clean your room?"

Paula also needed the world of words to slow down. She didn't need my constant interjections; she needed us both to sit in extended moments of silence. Paula moved in slow, precise motions and her personality matched this. She was serene and placid, completely different from me and the way I moved through the world. When she first came to see me for counseling, I was uncomfortable in the voiceless lull. I would lead with "Tell me about the time when..." and then wait agonizing minutes to hear her response. While she sat in complete quiet and calm, eyes downcast, my mind would race as I thought about what her response might be. I would play out our whole conversation in my mind before a word had come out of her mouth. Why couldn't she just answer in a timely manner?

But of course, the "timely manner" was of my own making.

"I have to see the word," Paula told me. "My mind is like a

filing cabinet. I see the word, then I have to find that word in the right file so that I can decipher what I see."

She explained that when I said the word *pen*, I might know which pen I was talking about, but Paula's file was full of different types of pens, like ballpoints, fountain pens, and markers. It took time for her to go through the file and select the correct pen.

Paula's explanation is backed up by science. The brain processes words in several regions, not just one. Neuroscientists are even mapping where specific word meanings are stored, making an "atlas" of the brain. They tend to be clustered together in groups. One region in the brain groups together kinship words, like *family*, *brother*, and *auntie*; another groups together *rake*, *shovel*, and *garden*. The human brain keeps words and concepts in filing cabinets, but some of us are running our auditory-processing files on an ultra-high-speed network while others are in analog, sending handwritten cards through the mail.

We all know what it is like not to be able to process what is being said. When we are distracted by our own thoughts, others' words might swirl around us but not really be heard. I have caught myself many times saying, "I am sorry, can you say that again? I wasn't really listening." It's not that I'm not interested; it's just that my mind is sometimes full and the words do not penetrate. While someone is telling you about their day, you might be thinking of what is on the shopping list. When someone is describing a great movie, you might be thinking of another movie you would like to talk about. And while we don't always process other people's words because we are lost in our own thoughts, we are an impatient bunch; we still expect everyone to listen to us and respond immediately to our requests.

When we ask someone to do something for us and they

don't respond within one and a half seconds, we are likely to ask again. But by doing so, we cut off the processing of the first request and are right back at the beginning of the auditory-processing journey. To make matters worse, when someone doesn't respond immediately, some of us begin to increase the number of words that we use:

"Hey, can you pass me that cup, please?" (One and a half seconds.) "I said, can you pass me the cup?" (One and a half seconds.) "How many times do I have to ask you? Can you pass me that cup?"

And now there are two questions that need responses. If we want to support auditory processing, we need to keep the number of words to a minimum.

Spoken words are impermanent and fleeting, and unless someone is truly listening, a lot of what is said can go in one ear and out the other. Whenever I hear a person say, "I told them," "I have said it a hundred times," or "I say it constantly," I am left wondering if their words are not being heard, not being retained. At these times, we need to rethink our own communication styles.

For many autistic people, words can be difficult to process, and the time it takes to translate them from sounds to meaning and back to sounds can be slower than it is for neurotypical people. And there's no rushing it; what's needed is just a bit of patience.

When I ask an autistic person a question, I sometimes count to thirty in my head. I may even count to forty-five. The response will always come. The silence can be uncomfortable, but it's mostly uncomfortable for me. Letting others know that there is no rush and that you are happy to sit comfortably until the answer comes is a far better way to communicate than firing off multiple questions.

They say silence is golden, and that is certainly true, because within the silence, the most value can often be found.

I asked Jimmy for a chat. I wanted to understand why he took so long to respond to my questions so I could figure out how I could support him while he thought about his answer.

"It just takes my brain longer, miss" was his very straightforward answer.

Together we worked out a plan. It was a plan that we would not disclose to anyone. It would be our secret.

Most kids are happy when a teacher is distracted; in fact, sometimes they will do whatever they can to distract a teacher from the work at hand. I used this to Jimmy's advantage.

"Jimmy, every time I ask you a question, I will not expect an answer from you until I have asked two more people. Got it? You, then two more people, then your answer."

He got it. We tried it out in class the next day. With the map of the world displayed for all the class to see, I started to fire off my questions.

"Jimmy, what is the capital of France?" I asked. Now it was up to me to play the distraction card. I dropped my pen (always a felt-tip), glanced out the window and made a comment about a cloud that looked like a turtle, or asked Jessica (who was always talking) to stop talking. I was the distractor to give Jimmy the time he needed. Then, as if I'd forgotten that I'd asked Jimmy a question, I continued with the other students.

"Beau, what is the capital of Iceland?"

"Hazel, what is the capital of Vietnam?"

And then back to Jimmy: "Oh, sorry, Jimmy, I didn't get your answer. What's the capital of France?"

"*Paris!*"

### PART III

# Empathizing

## Connecting and Belonging

My eight-year-old niece ran toward me from the water at the beach. Her normally long flowing hair was stuck to her shoulders, and her smile was way out in front of her flying feet. She was beaming, and it was so contagious she lit me up. Everything about her screamed *Life is good!*

"I'm playing with my friend," she chirped happily.

"Oh, is it a friend of yours from school?" I asked.

"Nooooo!" she sang.

"What's your friend's name?"

She shrugged her shoulders and turned away from me; I clearly had absolutely no idea how this friendship stuff worked.

Children never worry about names, titles, status, or job descriptions. They don't care which country you're from, what your gender is, or what color your skin is. They don't care if you can read or write or tie your shoes. They don't care about your bank balance, your politics, or to whom you pray. They're not concerned about what you did in the past or your plans for the future. The only thing they ever want to know is: "Wanna play with me?"

Children are brilliant in this way. No matter how different they may be from one another, they will try hard to find a way to connect. Children will grow fairy wings, create a universe with blocks, or fly to the moon in a cardboard box. Kids always find a way to build a bridge across a divide.

Humans are designed to connect with one another, and these interactions are said to be as important as food and water. When we are connected with other people, we feel that we're seen, listened to, and understood. It gives us the confidence to be our true selves.

This sense of connection is essential for mental health. Connection increases self-esteem and is a protective factor against loneliness and depression. We feel connected when our relationships are built on open communication, trust, and reciprocity, when we take the time to get to know one another's points of view and perspectives. We're connected when our relationships are authentic.

But if we hide or cover up parts of ourselves in an effort to create connection, is the relationship still genuine? Many autistic people feel the need to change their behavior in order to be included, but if they feel valued only for who they are when they behave in a neurotypical way, that's not connection — that's assimilation.

Inclusion isn't about a person having to fit in with the majority. Inclusion is the majority changing how they operate so that everyone feels heard and appreciated, safe and respected. Inclusion is when people's differences are lauded.

Billions of people share this planet, and we're rich in diversity of all kinds. But diversity presents challenges. Some people struggle to connect with others they view as different from themselves, whether because of neurology, politics, culture, or religion. But *no one* is exactly like anyone else. If we all operated on the logic of "I'm not interacting with them because they're not like me," no one would ever connect with anyone!

The incredible skill of empathy drives human connection. When we are empathetic, we don't need sameness — we just need to take the time to see things from others' perspectives and experiences. We all want to feel like we belong. When we do, it's in the knowledge that we are truly accepted with all of our uniqueness.

Maybe we should all start with "Do you want to play?" and take it from there.

# 20

# Bradley's Goggles

Bradley loved the outdoors and trampolines and monkey bars. At six years old, he would have been a worthy contestant for any race that involved climbing over, under, and through obstacles. He could have mastered the Spartan Race or Tough Mudder with the best of them. But today at the beach, Bradley was struggling with just one obstacle: he didn't have his goggles.

Bradley's family lived an hour's drive from the beach. His father, mother, and older sister had been planning this trip for weeks. That morning, they'd filled the car with towels and boogie boards and a picnic lunch to spend the day beside the water. It was going to be the perfect summer day. They had arrived and unpacked and set themselves up under their umbrella when Bradley asked a simple question:

"Where are my goggles?"

Bradley's goggles hadn't made it into the bag with the other beach gear, and things quickly fell apart. All the bags were rummaged through, clothes were turned inside out, and even the sandwiches, drinks, and apples in the ice cooler were inspected.

"I want my goggles," Bradley said.

"We can't drive home to get them, Bradley," his father said. "You'll just have to do without them."

Bradley said several times, with increasing insistence and volume, "*Go and get my goggles!*"

"No, Bradley, just calm down," his father replied with rising agitation.

But Bradley began to scream and cry, and his father reacted.

"Bradley, *stop it!*" he snapped. He was embarrassed that Bradley's meltdown was drawing attention. But Bradley couldn't stop. He screamed louder and threw his weight against his father and started kicking him.

"That's it!" his father barked and led the shrieking Bradley off the beach.

They weren't seeing the world through each other's eyes — with or without goggles.

We all want to be understood. We want other people to know what we're thinking and feeling without having to state these facts. We often expect that others, particularly those close to us, will know what we want and need and what our intentions are, and it's sometimes a shock when they don't.

Couples counseling provides a lot of insight into this desire for mind reading. Carol and Roy had been married for sixteen years when they came to see me. They both had very busy lives, working full-time jobs and raising three teenage children. Communication was often a struggle, and Carol stated that they were rarely on the same page.

"I'd just had a big day at work," Carol said, "and all I wanted to do was come home and have a shower, some dinner, and crash on the couch. When I walked in the door, I saw the house was trashed, and Roy and the kids were lounging around with their devices. No dinner had been prepared, no homework had been done, and the trash hadn't been taken out!"

Carol had confronted Roy. "Why can no one in this house ever lift a finger to help?" she yelled. "Why is everything always left up to me!"

She said that Roy walked out of the room without saying a thing, which only infuriated her more.

"Why did you walk away?" I asked him.

"Because Carol was upset," he replied. He turned to Carol. "You were yelling. You needed space."

"But I didn't want space," Carol said. "I wanted you to say, 'Darling, you must have had a hard day. Sit down and I will get you a glass of wine.'"

Roy looked shocked. "How was I supposed to know that?" he spluttered. "You didn't tell me!"

We want others to feel what we feel, see what we see, and understand our point of view without us having to articulate it. It's a big ask, but the fact that we understand that other people view the world differently and have their own unique attitudes, values, temperament, and tastes is one of our most incredible abilities.

When children are very young, they believe that everyone thinks and feels the same way they do. It is not until they are four or five years old that they start to understand that people view situations and experiences from different perspectives. This ability is a developmental milestone.

When my nephew was three years old, we played a game of hide-and-seek. It's a great game but often funny when played with a child who's not old enough to understand that you don't see the world as he sees it. I counted to ten, called, "Ready or not, here I come," and found my nephew in less than thirty seconds. He was lying in full view in front of the sofa with his head covered by a pillow. He thought that because he couldn't see me, I couldn't see him. He hadn't learned yet that we didn't share the same perspective.

Two years later I caught the same nephew in my kitchen with telltale signs all over his face that he had found the cookie stash.

"What have you been doing?" I asked.

"Nothing," he replied.

"Have you been eating my cookies?"

"No."

I laughed because he had finally done it! He was now old enough to know that we each had our own thoughts, and that we both saw that moment differently—and so he'd told a fib. He had made the developmental jump and realized that I hadn't been there when he'd had his hand in the cookie jar (although he had yet to learn how to hide the evidence).

When I first went to university, I studied history. I love history, because it's only the knowledge of the past that will allow us to change our future. I learned to consider the lived experiences of people from the past and see the world through their eyes. By doing so, I was able to consider what might have motivated them and what they might have felt. I could imagine the experiences of voiceless women on trial for witchcraft; the woeful standard of living in the Great Depression; and the bravery of those who set sail in wooden boats to explore unknown oceans.

By learning to think beyond my own experience, my own time, I was, little by little, able to shift away from simple judgments, ignore my own personal opinion, and think of how and why people acted and thought the way they did.

Empathy is the ability to imagine and feel what another person is experiencing. There are two types of empathy. Cognitive empathy is the ability to understand another person's thoughts and beliefs, and affective empathy (sometimes called emotional empathy) is the ability to understand a person's feelings and emotions and react to them.

Cognitive empathy means listening and then using your imagination. When someone tells you a story, you leave aside your own narrative and jump wholly and solely into theirs, building a picture of what it would be like if you were in their place.

A friend of mine recently missed out on getting into a university course and was desperately upset and disappointed. Instead of seeing this from my own perspective (I knew eventually my friend would be accepted into another course), I could sit in that moment of hurt and imagine how difficult it must have been to read the rejection e-mail.

We have the ability to cognitively empathize with the person in front of us, and, if that person tells us a tale about a cousin's best friend's sister's daughter, we are able to imagine what she would have experienced too. We might never have met the daughter, but we can pass through the intertwined relationships of space and time, put ourselves in that person's place, and try to see the world from her perspective. How incredible is that?

Affective empathy is when we feel another person's emotions and react appropriately. If we're with someone who is upset, we'll start to get upset too. When someone is rejoicing, we feel their elation.

When children see your tears and begin to cry too, they are practicing affective empathy. They may not have the capacity to understand the big picture or imagine why you are crying, but that doesn't mean they do not feel and react to your hurt. You demonstrate affective empathy when your friend tells you he's just had his heart broken, and you feel sad because your friend feels sad, even though you might not know any details of the breakup and you actually think he's better off without the other person.

Some people have an even balance of cognitive- and affective-empathy skills. Some have more of one type and less of the other. There's a myth that autistic people do not experience empathy, but nothing is further from reality. Many autistic people have difficulties with cognitive empathy but they have bucketloads of affective empathy.

Yusuf was the twelve-year-old autistic son of my close friend. He was a little boy with a big heart, but this wasn't always apparent. Yusuf understood electronics and was the person I turned to when I needed to link my new TV with my Wi-Fi network. He loved to pull things apart and see how they worked. His parents had even created a workshop for him in the garage. They'd visit recycling centers and collect broken toasters and stereos so that Yusuf wouldn't tinker with the perfectly good gadgets in the house. His knowledge of appliances was vast. The workings of people were a bit harder for him to grasp.

One steamy summer day, Yusuf's mom and I sat in their garden while Yusuf and his younger sister, Jamila, jumped on the trampoline. They'd turned it into a water park by placing a sprinkler near it so that it sprayed across them. They were having a great time until—like all siblings have done since time began—Yusuf started to call Jamila names.

"You're a bum," he said. "You're a dumb bum. You're the dumbest bum. You're the dumbest bum ever." He said it over and over again. Jamila got off the trampoline and ran to her mom in tears. Yusuf just kept jumping.

"Yusuf," his mom yelled. "That wasn't nice. Why do you think your sister is crying?"

Yusuf looked at his mother and crying sister. "I don't know," he replied. "I'm not Jamila."

This made sense: Yusuf was not Jamila, so how would he know her thoughts? He had difficulties with cognitive empathy, so he wasn't able to step into Jamila's shoes.

"Yusuf, your sister is sad. You've made her upset by calling her names. She is crying because you hurt her feelings," his mom said.

When she told him this, Yusuf climbed down from the trampoline and approached his sister. "Sorry, Jamila. Do you want a hug?" he offered. "Do you want to come back on the tramp and play with me? Sorry, Jamila, sorry."

Yusuf cared. He'd just needed to be told what emotions Jamila was having; he needed the information. Once he knew, he responded with affective empathy. He felt and showed sadness because Jamila was sad.

Autistic people can be highly empathetic and demonstrate deep levels of affective empathy, but sometimes they need a clear understanding of what a person is feeling first. Once this is understood, they can feel these feelings intensely and want to do all they can to alleviate another person's hurt and pain. In fact, some autistic people can be so overwhelmed with the emotions of others that they avoid social interactions altogether.

When people are highly empathetic, they feel other people's suffering deeply, and the depth of these emotions can sometimes be unbearable. Have you ever found it hard to cope with another person's emotional pain? When a friend is raging or in anguish, have you had difficulty handling it? Or when you watch the wars, riots, and famine on the TV news, do you lie awake at night pondering why some people don't have a roof over their heads, why some girls are not allowed to be educated, and why kids and teachers are being killed in school shootings?

Or do you watch, see, and hear, then let it go and move on to "What's for dinner?"

Hyper-empathy can suck people dry, but it can also be a source of great action. One of my favorite sayings by the Vietnamese Buddhist monk Thich Nhat Hanh is "Compassion is a verb." When I was in elementary school, I learned that a verb is a "doing" word. It is through empathy that we learn to be compassionate, and the best show of empathy is *doing* something to help and support others. There are countless stories of autistic people taking action because they feel others' suffering. They are fighting climate change, saving animals from extinction, discovering cures for diseases, and putting money in the hands of homeless people.

The more similar you are to someone, the easier it is to empathize, as your imagination doesn't have to make a great leap. But the skills of empathy are not truly tested by similarity; they are tested by difference. When you can envision, without judgment, the point of view of someone who differs from you in genetics, race, ethnicity, culture, place of birth, socioeconomic status, politics, age, religion, gender, sexuality, brain wiring, or experience, then you can tap into your power to be compassionate.

If neurotypical people are supposedly gifted with empathetic understanding, why aren't we better at empathizing with autistic people? Why are we not more open to and less judgmental of neurodivergence?

It doesn't take a lot, really. Just an open mind, an open heart, curiosity, and compassion. Being empathetic is the greatest adventure of life and brings the greatest rewards—from my perspective, anyway.

Bradley's dad escorted him to the car—not to drive him back to get his goggles but to give him some quiet time. While

Bradley sat in the car crying, his father circled it, walking off his frustration. Then his dad took a few deep breaths and went to Bradley.

"Why are your goggles so important, Bradley?" he asked.

"Daddy, you know that the sea hurts my eyes!" Bradley said between sobs. "You want me to have sore eyes and won't get my goggles!"

"Oh, mate." His father sighed. "I would *never* want you to have sore eyes. But if I drive all the way home to get your goggles, we wouldn't have any time at the beach. I just want us to have a fun day. Let's go, and I'll lift you up over all the waves so the water won't hurt you."

On hearing his father's loving, compassionate words, Bradley wiped away his tears and climbed out of the car. "Doesn't the water hurt you too, Daddy?" he asked.

# 21

# Alice's Dress

Alice looked like she had walked out of a 1950s fashion magazine. She was so glamorous in her flowing floral dresses with petticoats, perfect makeup, and scarves wrapped around her curled and primped hair, and she was covered in tattoos of pinup girls, cherries, and sparrows. I loved everything about her coolness. But something was amiss. Alice was too perfect. It was like she had stepped out of a photo shoot; every single component had been stylized to precision.

"I just don't feel like I'm myself most of the time," Alice told me when we met. "I'm faking being me." She based her look on various fashion codes. Alice showed me photos of herself from the past: as a punk in the early 1980s, hair gelled into a mohawk; as a Cyndi Lauper clone in the mid-1980s, swamped in beads and bracelets; and dressed in grunge in the 1990s.

"I'm never quite sure who I am," she said. "I take on a different character to blend in and always have."

Alice told me the name of the first girl she'd copied—Cindy Fullerton, who was the good girl in kindergarten. She told me that Cindy did everything right. She had good manners, was soft-spoken, and always had a slight smile on her face. She did whatever the teacher asked right away. She was given all the special jobs in class: feeding the fish and taking notes to the office. Mrs. Sullivan loved her and so did the other kids. Everyone wanted to play with Cindy, be Cindy's best friend, and have Cindy over for playdates.

"I just thought if I did everything the same way Cindy did, Mrs. Sullivan and the other kids would like me too," she said. "So, I acted like I *was* Cindy."

Alice could remember everyone she had modeled herself on. She listed the names of all the girls in grade school and high school. She was able to explain the small details of their voices and conversations and the way they interacted with one another. Alice said that she always knew she was different, but she never knew why. "I didn't want to be different, so I just tried hard to be the same as everyone else."

Alice had been mimicking her whole life, but she didn't have a name for what she was doing until she was diagnosed with autism at thirty-eight years old.

"Alice," I said, "it's called masking."

We all play many roles in life and wear many different hats. You may be a boss or an employee, a coach or a teammate, a teacher or a student. You may be all of these at once. And in all the roles you have to play, you present yourself in different ways. You change the way you act, dress, and speak depending on whom you are with. You have your phone voice. You clean yourself up and speak with rehearsed confidence at job interviews. You speak in a different "language" when you are with children versus when you are trying to impress a university professor. You don't fart or burp in the company of people you have just met, and you drop the swearing when you are with your grandparents. You might also present yourself differently in person and online, between reality and Instagram.

We all have times when we put on masks and "pretend" socially, when we do not feel like ourselves or comfortable in social situations. You know how awkward you feel when you go to a big event but don't know anyone? Maybe it's a massive party where you only know the birthday boy or one of those gala dinners with hundreds of people whom you've never met. Many people hate attending social events on their own. Extroverts who are skilled at breaking the ice can enter the space without care or concern, but the rest of us struggle until the ice has melted. (Or until we've had a glass of wine.)

Before social events like these, some people go into preparation mode. You might contemplate your outfit and change it several times. You might Google *What is neat/casual?* or *How fancy is black-tie?* (Very fancy.) You spend time thinking about how to start a conversation, practice some witty banter, and worry that you will be stuck standing alone in a sea of people with no one to talk to. The first ten or fifteen minutes after entering a roomful of people can be painful, but once you ease in, you can let your hair down. (Not literally — it's better not to literally let your hair down at a black-tie event.)

But for many neurodivergent people, every single social situation feels like those first uncomfortable minutes at a black-tie ball. No matter how big or small the group of people, for them, socializing can be distressing. And to cope with it and fit in, many autistic people learn to mask.

*Masking* describes how a person consciously or unconsciously hides aspects of themselves for self-protection when in social situations. Marginalized people who disguise parts of their identity in order to fit in are masking. Autistic people might go to great lengths to appear "non-autistic" and match the social norms that surround them. All of this takes consistent and deliberate effort. People might force themselves to make eye contact even if it hurts, copy the facial expressions or gestures of those around them, repress the need to stim, or imitate the dress style of their peers. They might even rehearse conversations and scripted responses to use with others.

My brother is an actor. He learns his lines and repeats them until they become his voice. He learns about the character's circumstances and where and in what time that character lives. His wardrobe will fit the role and he'll wear shoes that are not his own — he will literally walk in the shoes of another and will change his posture or gestures if the part demands it. Many autistic people who are socially motivated and seeking social acceptance, especially women, receive a late diagnosis because they are so adept at acting. They are masters of disguise. They have mimicked and masked their whole lives, playing a character and a role to perfection.

Kirsty was one of those women. When she came for her first appointment with me, she was dressed as if she worked in a corporate office. She wore a tailored skirt, a buttoned-up crisp white shirt, and polished low-heeled shoes. She was elegant and precise as she sat down, smoothing her skirt under her thighs, crossing her legs at her ankles, and folding her hands in her lap. At forty-two, Kirsty would have been a perfect fit at a big accounting firm, but we weren't doing tax returns — we were doing some counseling in a rural town where I sometimes wore flip-flops to work.

"I try to match my dress with the environment I'm in, like a type of uniform," she said as she looked around the room, which was filled with mismatched cushions on the floor and not a desk in sight. "I always dress for the occasion and mask in every situation."

Uniforms like Kirsty's can be useful. In the army, soldiers know one another's rank by their uniform, which means they always know what is expected of them. Soldiers would never wear combat fatigues or camouflage to a fancy dinner, nor would they wear formal dress in the field. For some people, a uniform makes it easier to know what to say and how to act—you just have to follow the rules of the dress code. Kirsty realized she was wearing the wrong uniform that day, and she was ruffled. She had clearly prepared to walk into a formal clinical environment, not one containing comfy couches and a coffee table.

Kirsty told me that she had started hiding bits of herself and copying others when she was bullied in school. "The other kids would tease me," she said. "They—mainly the girls—called me lots of names. They just knew I wasn't like them." So she watched and tried her hardest to fit in. She realized that the other girls didn't want to hear about the baby animals that she loved so much, so she learned to stop talking about them. And she laughed at their jokes, even if she didn't get the punch lines.

"I was so scared of being caught out. I was scared they wouldn't like me. Scared of being judged," Kirsty told me. "I had to pretend. It was for my own safety."

Autistic people mask their autistic characteristics out of fear of being excluded or not being understood. They're forced to hide their identities because of judgment and cruelty. When I think of people who are masking their autism, I'm reminded of others who have to hide their true selves. Many of my transgender clients talk of "hiding" their true gender and acting in the "gender role" that was assigned to them at birth. Clients who have yet to come out speak of concealing their sexual orientation, fearful of rejection or the reactions of others. Hiding their true identities has a major impact on their mental health and well-being.

Masking comes at a huge cost. We all know how tiring social events can be for some people. Many need time to relax afterward. They get home, pop the buttons open on their jeans, put their feet up on the coffee table, and sigh with relief. But there is a big difference between unwinding and exhaustion.

I recently took a red-eye overnight flight. I lost three hours crossing time zones and spent only two hours of that eight-hour flight dozing on and off on the tray in front of me, but I thought I was still quite sprightly. I ignored my aching body and my foggy brain and said, "I'm fine," when my sister-in-law asked if I wanted a nap after I arrived at her home in the morning. I sat on the couch to drink a cup of tea, and that's all I remember. I woke up two and a half hours later. That's exhaustion. It's not just being a little tired, a little lethargic; it takes away your ability to function. It causes dizziness and headaches. It interferes with your memory and makes you teary and irritable.

The fatigue that comes with masking is like getting on a red-eye every night. It takes a major toll on a person's mental health and can bring on autistic burnout. The emotional, mental, and physical exhaustion from masking can lead to a loss of both cognitive and communication skills. I have heard countless times from parents of autistic children that they are fine at school, but when they get home, they explode or don't engage for hours. That is because they have to run a marathon every day. They have suppressed and pretended and faked their way through. Recovering physically and mentally from a marathon can take weeks. Masking is, similarly, an endurance event, and people who have trained so hard to fit in can sometimes lose all sense of themselves.

"Many people say to me, 'But you don't look autistic,'" Lola said. "But I am. Sometimes I just don't quite know who I am, you know? Like, where does the autism begin and end?"

Lola was flamboyant, with multicolored hair and more earrings than I could count. She was an adventurer and thrillseeker who loved the heart-in-your-mouth feeling of parachuting and the hair-raising jolts of white-water rafting. Lola spoke in analogies. I loved spending time with her because I love analogies, particularly from someone with a quick-thinking and curious mind like Lola's. She used them constantly to describe her world, and she was always spot-on.

Lola had masked her whole life. When she was diagnosed, she said that the first question she asked herself was *Who am I, really?*

"I was like an undercover cop or a double agent who's been in character for too long and begins to wonder if they are themselves or the member of the gang or drug cartel they've been playing," she explained. "The lines blur—they no longer know who is real and who is the character. But there is always a breaking point when you just can't be undercover anymore."

Alice had spent a lifetime masking so that she could fit in. She had learned early on that it was "better" not to be herself, and she carried this notion into adulthood.

"I'd just pick a style that I knew I could wear," she explained. "I knew that if I had my costume on, I could find a way to fit in. My fashion is my camouflage. I can put on the clothes and makeup and just copy what I see around me. My whole life, I have just moved from one character to the next."

She described the anxiety that came with having to wear

each costume perfectly. Alice worried all the time that she would be discovered as a fraud, that those around her would know that she wasn't really a part of their tribe. We looked back at the photos of her past and she said, "I don't know if that was really me."

"Wouldn't you just like to be you, Alice?" I asked. "It sounds exhausting, playing a role all the time. Wouldn't you like to take the uniform and the mask off?"

"It does sound liberating to be just me," she said, "but it won't be easy to take all this protection off." She said she felt like the Man in the Iron Mask. She'd had it on her whole life, and it was suffocating. She wanted to rip it off. "But at the same time, I can't tear it off in one go," Alice said. "If you've been behind a mask for so long, you're sensitive. You have to pull it back slowly to reveal your true identity to the people you trust. A lot of raw skin and scabs have formed from a lifetime of hiding."

Many of us are unsure of ourselves in social situations — even the most confident people feel uncomfortable at times. And since we know this, shouldn't we be more welcoming of those who walk through life constantly feeling like this?

Imagine living your whole life pretending to be someone you're not and doing it so well that you confuse even yourself. Some autistic people say that masking their autism has given them opportunities in employment, friendships, and romantic relationships. When I hear this, it always saddens me. It upsets me not because they've been successful in these areas but because they've been successful in spite of themselves. Despite how far people have come in terms of awareness of diversity, many autistic people still need to act "not autistic" so that they're socially accepted by the wider community.

I'm left thinking that it's not the autistic community that needs to change — it's the rest of us.

# 22

# Sara's Dating Apps

Sara wanted a boyfriend—more than *anything*. "I want nothing else in life," she told me. In order to find one, she downloaded every available dating app. While some people's smartphones have social media, games, online banking, ridesharing, and streaming-service apps, Sara's apps consisted of Tinder, Bumble, Hinge, OkCupid, eHarmony, Zoosk, Badoo, Match.com, and Coffee Meets Bagel. Finding a boyfriend, for Sara, was serious business.

Sara was in her mid-twenties and worked three days a week at a fast-food restaurant, where she took orders, scooped fries, and poured sodas. She went to dinner at her mom's every Wednesday night and spent the rest of her time alone in her studio apartment, scrolling and swiping. Sara's home was filled with stuffed toys, pictures of kittens and puppies on the walls, and figurines of pink unicorns and fairies. It was magical and whimsical. But Sara had never had anyone other than family visit her apartment, and she never went out with others. Sara could not name a single friend.

"I have friends on Facebook and Instagram," she told me. "Heaps of them!"

Sara sent friend requests to hundreds of people—every

friend of a friend that she had on social media, people who were suggested by the algorithm, anyone linked to groups she was a part of, and anyone who had commented on the pages she liked. A lot of people accepted these requests — Sara actually did have hundreds of friends, except all of them were in cyberspace.

"I like their posts," she told me. "I like everyone's posts, and they like mine."

Sara's posts were all selfies in which she'd used filters to turn herself into a twinkling, glossy caricature. She glistened and sparkled and resembled the pictures and knickknacks in her home. Sara loved filters and thought they made her more beautiful and more likable than her real-life self.

But Sara wasn't interested in being liked by *everyone*. She wanted to be liked by one person, and she was making every effort to find that person through dating apps. Yet she had had no success in her virtual quest for love. Many people had swiped right or sent kisses, but after months and months (and hundreds of dollars), she'd had only one date.

"I don't know why it isn't working!" Sara complained. "I'm not picky; I don't even fill in my preferences apart from age. If I match with anyone, anyone at all, I just send them a message."

When she showed me the messages, the problem was clear:

Sara sent one message: *Hi!*

The person responded.

Sara sent three messages.

The person responded with one.

Sara sent eight messages.

No response.

Sara sent fifteen messages.

And another fifteen.

And another.

It was the same pattern every time. I wondered if Sara

understood the message being sent to her when she received no message at all.

"Sara, have you ever heard of reciprocation?" I asked.

Unrequited love! Songs, movies, poetry, and novels are filled with it. Shakespeare, Lionel Richie, *Love Actually,* and Taylor Swift have all expressed the pain of love that is not returned. Most of us experience this ache at some point in our lives. Unrequited love is the worst. It is like having the wind knocked out of you. It can hurt like hell—in fact, rejection actually registers as physical pain in the brain. It goes back to prehistoric days, when rejection by the tribe meant certain death. So these songs and tales of unrequited love are full of hundreds of thousands of years of despair.

"What will I do with all of this love?" Eddie asked me, sounding like the lyrics from a million songs. "Where do you put love if it is not wanted?"

The only outfit I had ever seen Eddie wearing was the unlikely combination of shorts and a woolen poncho. He was a man who believed in mysticism. He liked to dabble in peyote and ayahuasca and would relay to me the spiritual awakenings he had experienced by altering his state of consciousness. Eddie thought deeply about himself and his connection to the world and other people. He often shared psychedelic-sounding wisdom, like "The ego always comes from a place of emptiness; it is the essence that connects us all."

While Eddie was full of wonderful perspectives on life's many mysteries, relationships remained the most elusive to him. Eddie had come to see me for counseling due to a rejection that had sent him into depression—thoughts and feelings he did not know how to process.

"My heart isn't working properly anymore; it's sluggish and stabbing at the same time. How do I turn these feelings off?" he asked me. "Where does the love go when the person you so desperately want to give it to does not give it back?"

Unreciprocated love sucks.

*Reciprocity* is a word that I used to have trouble getting my tongue around. When I started giving training classes on relationships, sexuality, and disability, I practiced saying *reciprocity* over and over, just so I didn't mispronounce it in front of a crowd. I didn't want to get it wrong, because reciprocity is an essential component of the bond between people.

Reciprocation is the foundation of communication; communication in its simplest terms is about sharing. We want our interactions to be reciprocal in nature, but the ways people do this dance of giving and receiving can be vastly different.

Neurotypical people assume that when they talk to someone, that person will respond; when they ask a question, they expect that person to answer. If you're having a face-to-face conversation with someone, it would be quite awkward if you asked a question and were left hanging in silence, never receiving a reply. In the age of smartphones and texting and dating apps, though, things have become more confusing. Many people still expect others to respond to texts as quickly as if they were physically in the same room and they assume that others are available to chat at all times. This has taken reciprocal communication to a whole new level of complexity.

"I can see it," Libby told me. "I can see when it is delivered and when he's read it. I am so confused. If he has seen my message, why hasn't he responded?"

Libby was training to be a beautician and she practiced her skills on herself. She had thick, painted eyebrows that arched perfectly over her eyelash extensions. She was always in full makeup, with eye shadow that matched her outfits and lined lips that were plump and glossy. Libby could talk about how to maintain your eyebrows, how to apply eyeliner for a cat-eye, winged-eye, or reverse-cat-eye look, and how the shape of your face should determine your highlighting and contouring. I'm a person with limited cosmetic knowledge, so I learned a lot about makeup from her, but mostly she taught me about the overwhelming anxiety of unreciprocated and mixed messages in her on-again, off-again relationships in the digital age.

Libby had spent her formative years learning about reciprocation in neurotypical social interactions. She had been coached on greetings and had been explicitly taught "your turn, my turn" when it came to conversations. Libby was fully aware that neurotypical people expected a timely response when communicating in person, so she was perplexed that this expectation did not carry through to online interactions.

"I just don't understand," she told me. "We have been seeing each other for weeks. I really like him, but one day he sends me a lovely text and then I don't hear from him for five days. He never replies to my texts. But I can see when he is online, on Insta or Facebook or TikTok. I know he's seen my message and he's *ignoring* me."

Libby had become stuck and anxious. She was a runaway train, emotionally derailing in front of me; it was like I was watching pieces of her fall in slow motion. When there is no response, no reciprocation, it can feel like you are on a one-way track with no return. Libby admitted that when she didn't hear from him, she would scroll through his social media and reread all of his texts over and over, trying to find some hidden meaning.

"I just want to find anything that says he is thinking of me. *Anything*, Jodi!" she exclaimed, her voice cracking with anguish. "Why doesn't he just respond? Why isn't he following the communication rules?"

These expectations are deeply embedded in our social being.

We start learning to reciprocate as babies. A baby will cry to express its needs, and when the parent responds to these signals, that tiny baby begins its lifelong journey of back-and-forth interactions. Our understanding of reciprocity continues to build throughout childhood: We stack blocks together to build towers, throw and catch balls with partners, and learn how to take turns when playing games of snakes and ladders or snap. We learn to share our toys with the faith those toys will be returned. We develop the ability to socially initiate and respond and manage our "seesawing" interactions. You invite me for coffee; I invite you. You come and visit me at my place; I come and visit you. You lend me money or your lawn mower or a ladder; I do the same when you are in need. We alternate giving and receiving.

Differences in reciprocal communication are a component of an autism diagnosis; many autistic children do not develop reciprocity the same way their neurotypical peers do. Some people might not be able to maintain the back-and-forth of conversation; some might not be able to match an emotional exchange; and some might not understand how to take turns in a social interaction. Many of us have difficulty learning the art of reciprocation, but it's an essential component of cooperating and collaborating. It is in the mutual exchange that people benefit from one another.

That said, reciprocity is not about exchanging a cup of sugar for a cup of sugar. It's about knowing each other's needs and providing for them with equity, not necessarily equality. Sometimes we forget that what a person needs is different for everyone. We can demonstrate reciprocity by giving to people, but they might support us by giving back in a completely different way.

People often have disagreements about the distribution of household tasks. When you live with someone, you can get agitated when only one person is doing the dishes or taking out the trash. We often think every job should be taken in turns, but in some homes, turn-taking is not about creating a roster for whose night it is to cook or clean or change the kitty litter. Just this week, my mom mentioned that my dad likes to vacuum, but he hasn't cleaned a toilet bowl in years. She also recognizes that because she keeps the bathroom clean, she never has to sweep anything under the rug.

"We share everything equally, but I hate vacuuming and love a sparkling bathroom," she said. "Your dad is the opposite. Sometimes recognizing where your skills lie is the best way to support one another."

Reciprocity is not about a constant ebb and flow either. It cannot always be measured in an equal exchange of turn-taking. When someone is hurting or when a neurodivergent person does not demonstrate reciprocity in a typical way, the other person must be the better communicator. You cannot be the giver all the time, and neither should you be the taker, but there are times when you have to ramp up your "give" to support those who need it. Reciprocity is not always fifty-fifty. Sometimes it's sixty-forty, or eighty-twenty, or ninety-nine–one.

A person I care for deeply has been struggling with his mental health, and while I have been trying to throw joy at him, his cup is well and truly empty. It's hard to reciprocate joy and love when you are hurt or angry or confused by the world. But I remember that this person has stood by me at my lowest moments. He has thrown me a life buoy when I felt like my head was only just above water. That is the foundation of reciprocity. The support, care, and tenderness provided in the past creates a strong base. Reciprocity cannot be viewed in a single moment or a single day; it's a balance that happens over time. If the foundation of a relationship is solid, we're able to give more and expect less during the hard times. We can be each other's struts when our walls are wobbly.

We all want others to match what we give out socially and

emotionally. We want to feel that we are on the same page. We want our relationships to be like a well-coordinated dance: when one person steps forward, the other steps back, then vice versa. But we are not all great dancers. Some of us tread on each other's toes or have two left feet. Sometimes the better dancer needs to step up and take the lead to keep the dance flowing. After all, when it comes to reciprocity, it takes two to tango.

Long after Sara stopped seeing me for counseling, I saw her on the street. She was holding hands with a man wearing a tie-dyed rainbow shirt with the words HANG ON, LET ME OVERTHINK THIS emblazoned across his chest.

"Jodi!" Sara called, and we stopped to chat.

"This is Phoenix," she said, "my boyfriend." She twinkled and glistened like she had applied a real-life filter to herself.

We talked about their shopping for dinner; Phoenix was into cooking, and he was currently mastering Mexican food. He shared his best enchilada recipe with me, and we discussed whether or not cilantro should go in guacamole. And then we parted ways.

As I turned to look back at them, Sara turned too, and held up three fingers. I giggled.

"Three texts, Sara," I had said many moons ago. "Three, then wait." One for initiating, two for enthusiasm, three for requesting a response...then wait for reciprocation. These were the steps that Sara had practiced over and over again until she mastered them. We had spent hours practicing, months working out the intricacies of the back-and-forth: When to step in and when to step out. When to start and continue, and when to stop. When you are fifty-fifty, and when you have to give a little more or take a little less.

Sara had learned the choreography of reciprocity—and now she finally had her dance partner.

# 23

# Aaron's Honeymoon

Aaron and Brenda sat at opposite ends of the couch. This isn't uncommon in the first session of couples counseling. Brenda's crossed legs were pointing away from Aaron as if she wanted to make a quick dash in that direction, and he looked like he was in the front row of a class photo, stiff and upright, his hands folded in his lap. The armrests on either side were the only things holding them together.

You know how couples sometimes look like each other and dress similarly? These two were like that. Aaron and Brenda were both in jeans and white T-shirts and wore the same brand of high-top sneakers in different colors. They'd met online two years before and had been married for eight months. I was impressed that they were so proactive in seeking help; most couples don't seek support from a counselor until they are at a crisis point.

"When we first met, I was head over heels," Brenda began, "and everything about our relationship was magic. We loved all the same things and doing the same things." Brenda loved to cook and so did Aaron. Brenda loved to hike and so did Aaron. Brenda loved music festivals and so did Aaron. She said that she felt adored. He would bring her flowers and take her for candlelit dinners. Aaron had made her feel like she was the most special person alive.

"He told me early in our relationship that he was autistic, and I knew he didn't like to socialize, but that was fine with me," she said. "We had each other and we were happy. It may have been fast, but it was perfect, so when he proposed, of course I said yes."

But after they got married, the cracks began to show. Brenda said that now they never did anything together, and they couldn't communicate. They hadn't been out for dinner, hadn't been hiking, and hadn't gone to any music festivals for months. They weren't arguing—not beyond the usual day-to-day interactions about who was going to buy the bread or milk—they just rarely spoke.

"I've tried discussing the problems in our relationship, but Aaron avoids any conversation, so I gave up," she told me. "All of our problems are left unsolved."

Aaron sat in silence throughout Brenda's description of their marriage.

"What do you think about this, Aaron?" I asked.

"We don't need to do all of those romance things anymore," he said. "We're married. We've signed the certificate and that means we're committed to each other for the rest of our lives. I don't know what the problem is or why Brenda wants to keep talking about 'our relationship' all the time."

*Yep,* I thought, *looks like the honeymoon is over!*

The initial hit of attraction and the beginning of a romantic relationship is euphoric. You're giddy with excitement. You want to spend as much time as possible with this person, and all of your focus and energy is consumed by thoughts of your partner.

Science explains this love-drunk feeling. When you're falling in love, the brain releases large amounts of dopamine, which ignites feelings of reward and a sense of pleasure. It can stop you from eating and sleeping, make you feel literally crazy in love.

"I think about her all the time," Vanessa told me after she bounded into my office. She was almost floating. I'd never seen her like this before; she was usually surly and sullen, and she rarely smiled. She could be like a gray and overcast day, gloomy and sluggish. But not today. Today she was dazzling, and her words vibrated, all around the name Justine.

She spoke nonstop about Justine: What Justine did for work, what Justine liked to eat, where Justine had traveled last year. Justine was beautiful, Justine was funny, and Justine was a cat person too. Justine was the love of Vanessa's life.

"My family will think she's wonderful," this new Vanessa squealed, "and we'll go on a holiday together at the end of the year. And when we move in together, we'll be able to have two cats and cook vegetarian food every night." She told me her plans for how she would propose and what kind of wedding she thought they'd have.

"She sounds great!" I said. "How long have you been seeing her?"

"Oh, I just met her last night!"

We're all filled with optimism in the early stages of a relationship. Most of us know that to get from the first date to a committed relationship takes time and effort, but in these dazed beginnings, we tend to forget all the steps that must follow. The feelings of attraction and engaging in a special interest are much the same, and for some autistic people, this new and exciting person can become their sole focus. Some autistic people, like Vanessa, become utterly infatuated and throw the cautious pace of relationship development to the wind.

It's true that when you're in this energized, dizzy stage, you want to do everything you can to impress the other person and present your best self. But you can't operate in this sustained adrenaline rush forever, and of course, your raw and real self has to come out eventually.

During those first weeks or months, you also see your new love as the perfect person. But for a relationship to settle and have longevity, you need to love that person's whole self, including all the flaws and annoying habits. You may initially see this person shaded in brilliance, but eventually the rose-colored glasses come off. And then you see it: the imperfection. Maybe your new love eats with her mouth open, talks through a movie (or can never keep track of the plot), and doesn't clean the sink after brushing her teeth, and that once-cute snore now keeps you awake all night. Suddenly you go from being one loved-up entity to two whole humans again, and you need to start communicating your own wants, needs, and desires.

People come with differences of opinion and different ways of expressing themselves. Because we all perceive and communicate differently, it's only natural that we misunderstand each other. Learning how to address issues together is therefore essential if you want to be in an intimate union with someone.

My sister and brother-in-law have a loving relationship. They support each other and laugh at each other's jokes and problem-solve together. One morning I was watching them as they sat at the dining table, drinking tea and doing the crossword.

"You two communicate really well," I commented.

"Not every day," my sister replied. "Not all the time, but

even if we have trouble communicating today, we'll find a way to do it better tomorrow. It's taken a lot of practice."

She threw out this line flippantly, but I heard it with the reverence it deserved.

People in healthy relationships know how to communicate when their differences give rise to conflict. But conflict doesn't have to be a dirty word as long as it is followed by an even more important one: resolution.

Communicating when the road is rocky takes the highest level of social skills that we humans possess. For autistic people who have difficulties with social interaction, these hard conversations can be excruciating, particularly when they involve a lot of emotion. Autistic people process and interpret verbal and nonverbal communication differently, and they might have trouble expressing their emotions or identifying emotions in others. As a result, they might become overwhelmed by tough conversations—even more so than neurotypical people—which can cause them to be reactive or try to dodge these discussions altogether.

Petra struggled with this type of interaction, and her partner said that unless they sought help, their relationship could not continue. Petra loved her partner and was highly motivated to make it work. But she didn't know how to communicate in a productive way.

"I cause a lot of hurt," Petra told me. "I don't mean to, but when Gilles brings up problems, I get frightened. I think he's angry at me, so I lash out, and this always goes horribly wrong."

As he listened to her talk, Gilles placed his hand on her knee. "I know that Petra loves me," he said kindly, "but when we have any problem, when even one tiny thing goes wrong, Petra thinks I am criticizing her. When I try to talk about it, she misinterprets my intent and my tone."

Petra perceived any difficult conversations as a threat to their relationship, so she became defensive. Because of the way her brain was wired, when Petra was upset, she was unable to process Gilles's words. Her auditory processing became overwhelmed, and she would often react by going on the attack. She would blame Gilles for the problem, make excuses, or bring up Gilles's past mistakes.

We can all become defensive when we feel we are being criticized, but this loop of communication prevents us from resolving the issues. In fact, it makes matters worse. With Gilles's help, they established some rules for communicating at these times. Rather than just bringing up issues out of the blue, Gilles learned to schedule time with Petra to talk about them and never when they were rushed or tired. They agreed to stick to the immediate problem and not bring up past issues. If Petra became emotional, Gilles or Petra would say, "Need a break" — not as a question but as a statement for them both. Once the negative emotions passed, they'd commit to coming back to continue their conversation. And Petra learned that a good relationship isn't based on an absence of issues or fights but on knowing how to fight.

Rather than avoiding conflict, we need to learn how to fight fair. In healthy relationships, fights should not be about who wins—they should be about building a stronger team. But we need to remember that not everyone wants to jump into this ring.

Some people have no interest in moving into the conflict stage of a relationship. Bryson, a force of nature with a swagger and a big cheeky grin, would throw in the towel at the first disagreement. When the bubble popped and a love interest shifted into a phase of negotiation, Bryson was out. He was up-front in his attitude about relationships; by choice, he'd never had one that lasted more than a few months. Once the thrill was gone, he was gone too.

"That's love, that feeling of rush and excitement," he told me. "Humdrum day-to-day reality? That's such a downer. I just want the feeling of when we first met, that loved-up buzz."

So Bryson moved from one person to the next at lightning speed. And that was okay—as long as the people he was loving and leaving understood that Bryson's interest was a hot fire that would extinguish fast. Long-term relationships are not for everyone. Bryson and I spent a lot of time talking about how he could best communicate this to others so he didn't leave burned and broken hearts in his wake.

When I was young, I had a vision of how my life would be. I would have a long-term partner, a happy home (in my mind, this was a farm with chickens), and a crew of children, five or maybe six. I'd read the fairy tales and watched all the rom-coms and held the belief that everyone had a soul mate, that one perfect person. It was a big dream, and while the egg collecting and the six kids might not be on everyone's bucket list, a lot of us do hope for a life partner. The "one forever love" didn't become a reality for me. I've loved more than one person with a big open heart, and I've been deeply loved in return. But it took me a while to recognize that not being with one person forever and a day was not a failure.

*Cinderella* and *Pretty Woman* taught me (and millions of others) that having one true love equals "success." Society promotes the idea that people need to be coupled to find happiness. We have to change this narrative, because a good life is not about being in a romantic relationship—it's about *having* good relationships. With a partner, sure, but also with friends and family.

We also need to dispense with "They lived happily ever

after." Relationships cannot be perpetually happy. There are ups and downs and good moments and bad—sometimes very bad. There's a saying that people often fall in and out of love in long-term relationships. There are times of deep connection, but there are also times of simple coexistence. There are times of flowers and champagne and times of bread and milk. But each stage in a relationship takes effort, and both parties need to work together. Each of us brings something unique to a relationship, and we need to strive to understand and accept each other's differences. Because we are constantly evolving, this work never stops.

One couple I met while traveling told me that they had the perfect relationship. *No way,* I thought. No relationship is perfect. People have misunderstandings and arguments. They have different wants and needs. They can be frustrated or just plain bored with each other. I asked them what made their relationship perfect.

"No matter what, we have each other's back," they replied. "No matter what hardships or obstacles our relationship faces, we're going to be there for each other."

Now that I think of it, that sounds pretty perfect to me.

When the honeymoon period is over, we have to discard our expectations of what we think the relationship should be and start seeing it for what it really is.

Aaron was besotted with Brenda and wanted to spend the rest of his life with her. Once they happily signed on the dotted line, he felt that the rest was "ever after." He didn't grasp that this was not the end—it was the beginning. He didn't realize that when the two of you drive off into the sunset, you still have to regularly stop for fuel and to put air in the tires.

"When we first met, Brenda was like a special interest," he

gushed. "I wanted to know everything about her, wanted to do whatever she wanted to do. I couldn't stop thinking about her." He explained that once they were committed for life, he felt secure, and in this security, he no longer thought about her all the time. He didn't understand why Brenda wanted to talk about their relationship constantly. He didn't know he had to keep working at it.

Brenda learned a lot too. She'd thought autistic meant "not social" and she did a deep dive to educate herself. They both committed to learn about each other's communication style and the ways in which they expressed and understood emotions. They scheduled a time each week to discuss their relationship, and they also scheduled date nights, time together, and time alone. They talked about how they wanted to be loved and how they showed love.

Six months after Brenda and Aaron first came to see me, they were still sitting on the couch. But now they were both in the middle, wearing their matching high-tops, side by side.

# 24

# Harry's Trench

When Harry first entered my room, his hoodie was pulled down and his bangs hung so low they obscured his face. He was like a caged animal in an unknown space with a stranger. A stranger he was wary of.

Have you ever brought a new puppy or kitten home, put it down for the first time, and watched it scope out the room? It looks in all the corners and sniffs out the safe spots, and if you give it all the time it needs, it approaches you when it's ready. People do this too. If they don't feel safe, they might inspect a new environment, work out the escape routes, and look for places where they are able to retreat.

Harry did this the first day I met him and for many days after. He had lived in the foster-care system since he was six. Now fifteen, he was tall and gangly with long oily hair and a face covered in teenage acne. He had been referred to me because he needed to complete a victim's statement for the abuse he had experienced and witnessed in his childhood home as well as in multiple foster placements.

He was initially funded for five hours of counseling to complete the victim's statement. *Five hours!* Think of the people you have spent only five hours with. Is this enough time for you to feel you could tell them all of your hurt and shame?

Harry moved with the lumbering gait of a teenage boy whose extremities had outgrown his body. And he moved all the time. At our first appointment, he said almost nothing. He just paced the room.

"I don't want to be here" was all he offered. "So I'm not talking."

"That's okay," I said, and then it was the longest fifty minutes of my life. I sat while Harry walked and surveyed. He lifted things and turned them over. He pulled books from shelves and flicked through pages and almost wore a hole in the carpet as he paced back and forth. I felt like I was in a therapy session in *Good Will Hunting*. My thoughts darted about. *Should I pick up some paper and draw? No, then he will think I don't care. Should I just talk about nothingness? No, then he will think I don't want to listen.* I sat in complete silence and didn't move a muscle; we were yin and yang in motion and stillness.

When I saw the clock on the wall indicate minute fifty, I nearly cried out in relief. "Well, you did it, Harry." I exhaled. "You made it through and you didn't walk out! That's pretty impressive in my book."

Harry darted out of the room without a goodbye or a glance in my direction. I immediately e-mailed the department and told them I needed way more than five hours. I may have added a few choice words concerning expectations and outcomes, so they allocated me the time.

Over the coming weeks, I had to learn my way around Harry, as he startled easily. I cursed myself every time I made him jump. If I approached him from behind without announcing myself, he jumped. But if I announced myself while I was too close—"Hey, Harry"—he also jumped. I once touched his arm and he reacted as if I had thrown acid on him. He tried to push me away with his words: "I'm bored." "You're so boring." "How stupid are you?" He would sulk and sigh and create chaos in the space, ripping paper into tiny pieces and throwing it like confetti. (The vacuum always got a good workout after Harry came for an appointment.) He knew what we were there to do, he knew what was expected of him, but there was no way that Harry was going to tell *me* anything.

I needed to be patient until Harry was ready to tell me his story.

I've always been fascinated by people who tattoo words on their skin. It's a brave thing to do. Out of all the words and phrases that exist, which would you choose to mark your body with permanently, with no regrets?

My brother has the word *patience* tattooed on his forearm. It's a beautiful word. He told me that it's his favorite, but it's also a constant reminder that there is no need to rush through life. Remembering this isn't easy, as we live in a time when things are immediately at our fingertips. We can zap food in seconds in the microwave or order it on our phones and have it delivered. We can binge-watch a whole TV series without having to sit on the cliff-hanger for a week until the next episode, and in an instant, we can chat to anyone on the planet on Face-Time, Zoom, or Skype. Being able to get immediate results means that any delay in gratification can be difficult.

We want to achieve things quickly because we're living in a fast-paced, hectic world, and many of us are multitasking and juggling a lot at once. When you ask another person, "How are you?" have you noticed that a common response is "Busy"? Why do we equate busyness with success? Do we really need to be productive every second? When was the last time you just sat on the couch, looked off into space, and daydreamed? Many of us are unfamiliar with the art of doing nothing. But doing nothing, being able to sit still and be right there in the moment, teaches us patience.

When I was running support groups for parents of young autistic children in early-intervention settings, we would discuss how important it is to play with kids. But lots of adults don't actually know how to play. A lot of us pretend to play, but we're not really present. We might be building Legos with a toddler, but at the same time our heads are constantly buzzing with what we have to do next. When children play, they're thinking of nothing else but what's in front of them. They're in the moment, and play is all they think about. During these support groups, I would ask the parents to have a go at just "doing" with their kids — just play and try not to jump into the future in their own heads.

A week after I proposed this challenge, one mom returned to the group with her story. She explained that her son always wanted to read at least three books every night and often pushed for more. She would lie next to him in bed and read out loud, but she was always hoping he would go to sleep quickly so she could have some time for herself or get jobs done around the house.

"But last night, I decided just to read," the mom said. She committed to not running through her checklist, just to lie down and get lost in the books. "It was amazing. I really got into the stories and put on voices and asked him lots of questions. And do you know what he said to me?" In the middle of reading, her son turned to her and asked, "Why are you so happy tonight, Mommy?"

Being patient is good for you; it's linked to feelings of happiness and relieves stress. Being impatient can have a negative impact on both you and others. Other people know when you're impatient. You can pretend as much as you like, but impatience oozes out. Patience comes across as easygoing and levelheaded calmness; impatience comes across as frustration.

I'm not a very patient person when it comes to myself. The words *patient* and *patience* are from the same root word meaning "to calmly endure," but I'm terrible at calmly enduring when I *am* the patient.

Several years ago, I hurt my back and had to spend days in the hospital, then weeks lying on my stomach, walking on crutches, and learning how to get my right leg back online with the rest of my limbs. I was a dreadful patient. I'd lost control over my own body and I needed to recover immediately. I was frustrated and short-tempered, and I wanted results *now*. I expected to bounce back quickly. So I pushed my body beyond its capacity and caused more setbacks and more pain.

Finally, I was told it would take two years before I would know the extent of the permanent damage, and I realized I had to accept my situation. Two years was a long way away—far too long to live in constant, impatient frustration. Rather than looking into the future, I needed to shift my assumptions and learn to celebrate the small day-to-day improvements. I needed to let go of my thoughts of *I should be better by now.*

There are a lot of *shoulds* embedded in our impatience with ourselves and others. We may think another person should be doing it *this* quickly or should be doing it *this* way; the person should be completing it at *this* time and at *this* pace, and the outcome should look like *this*. Just this morning, I watched a man huff and puff while he waited for the barista to get his coffee. "What's taking you so long?" he bluntly asked her. "I need to get to work!" He had arrived and ordered after me and three other people who were also eager for their caffeine hits, but he expected that the milk should be frothed and his cappuccino ready on his schedule. When people don't do things the way we think they should, we get impatient. But we don't all do things in the same way at the same time.

Many autistic people live in other people's *shoulds*—that they *should* be moving through the world in a neurotypical way. If we expect autistic people to be typical, then they are set up to fail. Our capacity to be patient shifts when we see other people as different from ourselves, when we adjust our time frames, our expectations, and our views of what the outcome must be. Impatience is based on only one perspective—one's own. When we are patient with others, we turn our thoughts away from our own needs and accept that we don't all conform to one way of thinking.

Patience lies within us. We can't control every situation and we cannot make other people do it our way on our time. When we start to feel irritated, when things are not going the way we planned or the way we want, this is when we need to practice patience.

And patience is a practice.

"I'll never ask you to tell me, but I'm ready when you're ready," I finally said to Harry after weeks.

Harry and I had spent months not talking. Well, we started talking a lot, but never about the things that mattered—the things that the department needed to hear.

Harry had an interest in military history. He was particularly fascinated by World War II and the Holocaust. I remembered when I first learned about this moment in history, and I had been fascinated too. I had devoured books about the war and read *The Diary of Anne Frank* too many times to count. Harry and I talked about it often, and he was always perplexed:

"How could people do that to other people?" he once asked me. I had no answer for that one.

And because he needed to move, that's what we did. We'd go to the sports field and kick a soccer ball, and he'd try to teach me the fine art of the Maradona turn; I never mastered it. We'd walk to the park and swing on the swings; he's the only person who has ever convinced me to jump from a swing in flight. When it rained, I introduced him to yoga, and both of us rolled around on mats on the floor.

One day after we'd been meeting for about a year, as he paced and I sat, we discussed an upcoming day of remembrance for all the people who had served and died in wars.

"You're a bit like a person who has been in a war zone, Harry," I stated, almost talking to myself. I told him that many people who had been at war had something called hypervigilance. People had dug themselves trenches and lived in these holes in the mud and rain. They'd lived in constant fear, frightened to lift their heads. They'd spent so long watching for danger and knowing that at any time they could be attacked that their brains couldn't stop thinking like that even when they got home, even when they were safe.

As I spoke, Harry came and sat down beside me. He had never done this before. I kept talking. "We all need places where we feel safe and people we feel safe with," I told him. "When we feel safe, we can relax and feel confident." And as I rambled on, Harry leaned toward me and rested his shoulder against mine. I tried hard to hide my joy and not make a big deal out of it. Harry was touching me for the first time.

A year after Harry first leaned against me, he was finally ready for us to write the victim's statement together.

"I'm not going to look at you when I write this all down," I said. "I'm not going to show any emotions on my face at all.

That's not because I don't care about what you are going to say; I just know that it is going to be hard for you to say it, and it might be hard for me to hear."

The stories were horrific, and inside I was screaming at what this beautiful young person had been through. At what people could do to other people.

It took two years for Harry to tell me his story. This wasn't an easy time for me. I had to shift my expectations and *shoulds* to match Harry's. It was frustrating, but all I could do was calmly hold on. And in those two years, Harry found the faith and knowledge that I would sit, solid and secure as a rock, so he could share all of his vulnerability. In patience, Harry found safety.

Sometimes what we need is patience—a lot of it. Patience can be the kindest gift that we can offer each other.

# 25

# Andre's Concerto

Andre had a man bun. I thought he was maybe following a fashion, but he quickly told me that it was because he hated having his hair cut (the scissors hurt his hair) and he hated having hair in his eyes.

"I'm also quite lazy," he said. He told me he normally just rolled out of bed and put on the clothes he found on the floor. His T-shirt and button-up were always wrinkled, his cargo pants were scrunched, and he wore socks that not only didn't match but were *completely* mismatched—for instance, one red and one green covered with pineapples.

His home had the same look of abandon. Walking into his apartment for the first time, I felt that either Andre was on the verge of a great invention or that he was lost in his own chaos. The living room had no couch, no coffee table, and no TV. Instead, it was a music studio. There was an upright piano, a keyboard, several guitars, a mandolin, and all manner of percussion instruments as well as cables, amps, headphones, and computers. And sheet music was everywhere. It covered the floor and surfaces like leaves at the end of fall, landing wherever they had been blown.

Andre was a brilliant musician. He was a composer and spent all day and all night with his instruments. He didn't socialize with anyone, didn't go anywhere. Family members dropped in on occasion, but other than that, Andre was alone. It was just Andre and his instruments. Every day, for months and months at a time. I had been called in because people were concerned about his lack of social interaction.

I was worried too. He was so isolated, had no friends, and spent all his time all by himself. He was living my worst nightmare. "You must be lonely, Andre," I once commented, thinking about how much I loved people and couldn't live without them.

"I don't know what you mean," he replied. "Why would I be lonely?"

Being alone and being lonely are two different things. *Lonely* is an emotion, a feeling of isolation or that something is missing. *Alone* is all about solitude, and it can give people a sense of peace. Some people love being alone and rejoice in their own company, while others are lonely and yearn to connect with others. Aloneness can bring contentment, whereas contentment will never be found in loneliness.

My neighbor Arthur lived on our street for thirty-five years. When he first arrived, there was a sheep pasture across from his house; that's where my house now stands. When I became Arthur's neighbor, every time he saw me, he would wander across the potholed road that separated us to tell me what the weather was going to do or give me gardening advice.

"You should cut down those palms, sweetheart," he would instruct me. "They're terrible things, dropping all of those fronds. A complete menace!"

Arthur had lived alone since his wife died. "I lost my

darling seventeen years ago," he told me, his eyes cast down. I could hear the desolation in Arthur's voice, so I began dropping off leftovers, and I'd stop by to ask him for an egg or to borrow his rake. I took note of the pattern of his day—what time his blinds went up in the morning and when his lights went out at night. I knew his sheets went out on Tuesday and that he mowed the lawn on Saturday. I knew that when Arthur's routine was off, something was not quite right, and when that happened, I'd go check on him.

"Getting old can be lonely," he said to me one day not long before he went to join his darling. "Sometimes you're the only person I speak to all week." Arthur died at the ripe old age of ninety-two. I still miss him.

There is a longing in loneliness, a deep desire and need for connection and companionship. Loneliness has a major impact on a person's mental and physical health and has been linked to an increased risk of cardiac disease; it is, literally, a disease of the heart.

All of us experience that terrible feeling of loneliness in our own unique way. Most of us know what it feels like to be left out of a game at recess, start college, move to a new town, or retire from a job and lose day-to-day contact with others. These bouts of transient loneliness subside when people meet or reconnect with others. Chronic loneliness, however, is the prolonged feeling that there is no conceivable end in sight to this agonizing emotion. It is awful and gnaws away at the human spirit.

When we think of loneliness, we associate it with being alone, but you don't have to be sitting in a dark room without another soul to feel it. One of my clients once confided to me that they felt lonely in their own bed while sleeping right next to another person.

"How can that be?" they asked me. "I can hear the rise and fall of their breathing and the rumbling of their stomach, yet I lie awake and feel utterly cut off from everyone."

It's strange to think we can be lonely in the presence of the person we are closest to, but even in the strongest of relationships, one or both people can drift apart or feel estranged for a time. People can feel lonely even when surrounded by a whole community or in a roomful of people, a school filled with students, or a city filled with millions. A person can feel like a wallflower.

"They never knew I was there. I was forgotten," Daisy said.

Daisy, at twenty-two, smelled of cigarettes and flowery deodorant. She was a paradox in this and many other ways. She was vivacious yet listless, courageous yet timid, confident yet afraid. She was beautiful, but she couldn't see her own beauty.

It took years for Daisy to tell me her story—years of appointments to help her navigate an autism diagnosis that she had received in adolescence. When Daisy was first diagnosed, she did not want to be labeled. She said that she had always felt like an outsider and that being autistic just made her feel even more different. She wanted so desperately to belong.

When I asked Daisy about her experiences at school and what that time was like for her, she would laugh and simply say, "It was shit." I knew the story would come; I knew if I was patient enough, the story would not be masked by laughter. When she finally told me, it hit with the force of a tsunami.

"I was like a speck of dust," she stated. "I moved to a new school when I was twelve, and it was terrible. No one spoke to me. No one introduced themselves. No one invited me to sit with them or to play. Everyone knew each other and I couldn't fit in. I was an outcast, a social pariah. They knew I was different, and they rejected me. No one wanted me."

She explained that she spent nearly every day of that first year of school in an office near the reception desk. The room housed the school stationery and photocopier. She would leave class and go there, or she'd act up in class until she was kicked out and then sneak in there. She spent every recess and lunch in this space.

"It was the safest place, because if I sat there, I was alone," she said.

Daisy told me that there was a gap between the filing cabinets, and sometimes she would jam herself into that gap and fall asleep. I pictured children hiding under their beds, in closets, or under their blankets during a thunderstorm. I felt the fear and the isolation. "But didn't the staff know?" I asked. "Didn't anyone come to look for you? To help you?"

"No, I was invisible and forgotten." The tears welled and spilled without stopping. "I was lonely. I was so, so lonely," she said, weeping. And then she heaved a breath and began to howl.

I felt my heart crack for the girl who was reliving the depths of this misery ten years later. I felt the lump in my throat form as I watched the woman sitting across from me, filling tissues with tears and pain.

Four years after she started at that school, she was given an autism diagnosis. "And do you know what the worst bit about that was?" she asked me. "Every single person, every doctor and psychologist and occupational therapist and counselor and every person on the mental-health wards, always asked the same question: 'Do you have any friends?'" This was a constant and stark reminder that she had had none.

We all want to feel that we belong, that we are connected. My number one fear has always been loneliness, but I don't mind having time alone.

We live in a world where being an extrovert is prized. If you spend Friday night at home enjoying a book and a glass of red wine, there must be something wrong with you, right? But some people love time on their own and never once feel lonely in their own company. Some people don't need constant interaction with others to feel fulfilled, and they use this time to recharge their batteries. Others just love their own space.

A gregarious friend of mine told me that he is left exhausted after interacting with people. I was startled by this because he has a big, bold, life-of-the-party personality.

"Oh, I love spending time with people, but not a long time," he said. "I'm a homebody, really. That's where I feel most comfortable."

Being alone is exactly what some people need for their well-being. In fact, we all need it occasionally. "Yay, I got to go to the toilet by myself for the first time in months," new parents say. "I love a bath so I can shut the door and forget the world," says anyone who wants to escape a busy household.

While loneliness is linked to poor health, solitude is linked to improved mental health. Solitude allows you to feel centered and grounded. It's only in moments of solitude that you give yourself the gift of reflection, contemplation, and creativity. Sometimes you just need time alone to thoroughly connect with yourself.

Spending time alone can be a choice. Loneliness is not. When people are lonely, life feels empty. Loneliness makes people feel unwanted and unloved. And the best way to solve this seemingly unsolvable problem is to look around you and consider the people who might need a little more connection in their lives. Sometimes you need to reach out and check in. Sometimes you need to ask, "Are you okay on your own, or do you want some company?"

Arthur and I reached out to each other.

"If I disappear, do you think anyone will notice, sweetheart?" Arthur once asked me. "If I died, would my body be left for days?"

"No way," I replied. "Not on my watch, Arthur!"

Many years after I met Andre, he sent me a message and asked if I would like to attend his graduation from the conservatory of music.

I entered the auditorium and took a seat among hundreds and hundreds of people. The graduating students performed brilliantly and I enjoyed it, but I was there for one person and one person only. When Andre walked across the stage and took a seat at the piano, he was poised and calm—but his man bun was still a mass of unkempt hair.

Silence fell as Andre began to play. The music started slow and deep and then moved to joyful and brisk.

I could see a man to my left slowly tapping his finger to the music on his pants leg and the person to my right tapping a foot. Then the music shifted and pulled me away from the people beside me. Sometimes I felt like I was in the strong rapids of a river and other times in the cool stillness of a water hole. I imagined all of this as Andre moved his fingers up and down the keys. The music he wrote and was now performing was haunting and beautiful.

I thought about when I entered the library at Trinity College in Dublin and saw the number of books there. How could there be so many books and so little time to read them? And I thought of the time I saw one of Monet's water lily paintings; I was transported into his garden and filled with a sense of calm and peace. I was brought to tears in both of these moments, flooded with feelings of awe, but I had not met the writers of those books or the painter who had brought me so much pleasure.

I closed my eyes and listened to Andre. And then I felt it; my heart swelled and all the hairs on my arms stood straight up and the tears began to well. I turned to my left and saw the man next to me wiping away a tear under his eye with his finger. I turned to my right and saw gentle, unashamed tears running down the cheeks of the person beside me.

Loneliness and being alone are different experiences for all of us. Some people need others each and every day and dislike being on their own. Some need just one or two like-minded people to feel fulfilled. And some people, like Andre, enjoy being alone but can create a connection with hundreds of people without ever having been introduced.

# 26

# Malik's Echidna

"Online grocery shopping is the best thing ever invented," Malik said. "Actually, all online shopping—you can buy everything and never have to speak to a person, let alone see them!"

Malik was a cyberspace whiz. His living room was set up with multiple computer monitors, some with split screens. He could game across two displays, have computer code up on a third, and be scouring the internet on a fourth, all at the same time.

Malik was a good-looking guy with the chiseled features of a Michelangelo sculpture, but he didn't see himself the way I saw him. "I'm ugly" was how he described himself. He followed this with a list of cruel self-critiques, among them that he was skinny, weak, and worthless. He thought this was how other people saw him too.

Malik lived alone and rarely left the house. He never made or answered phone calls; it was texting or nothing. He didn't like to talk to strangers or be too close to them. He didn't like going to the store or the bank or even sitting in a waiting room. He always messaged me before coming to an appointment to make sure no one else was in the office. People made Malik's palms sweat and his legs shake. Social interactions made him anxious.

"I can feel people appraising me, examining me," he told me. "I hate it. People will size me up and decide if they like me or not within the first seven seconds. It's wrong. Humans are so judgmental."

No matter where he went, Malik believed people were looking at him with a critical eye. He imagined that each and every person he met was looking for the worst in him and saw only flaws and faults. He thought that everyone saw themselves as superior to him, and this made him feel insignificant. Malik was frightened of the way that other people made him feel; their judgment scared him.

Malik disliked people, but he *loved* animals. He could spout all sorts of facts about mammals, birds, and reptiles. He wasn't so into fish or amphibians, but he'd still be the guy you'd want on your team when an animal question popped up at trivia night. He was particularly fond of Australian marsupials and monotremes, and when he spoke of them, his face brimmed with confidence.

"One day I'd like to do a wildlife-rescue course so I can look after native animals at home," Malik once dropped into our conversation.

I nearly fell off my chair. Malik, the man who loathed people, was willing to be with people if it meant he could spend more time with animals.

"I've always wanted to do one of those courses too!" I lied.

In Australia, we're constantly surrounded by all kinds of wonderful wildlife. This is especially true if you live outside the big cities, which Malik and I both did. Occasionally people find a hurt wallaby or a kookaburra with a broken wing by the side of the road, but most of them don't have a clue how to help it. Thankfully, some nature-loving people train as volunteer wildlife rescuers and are called in to help the public when they find a sick or injured animal. The rescuers then take the animal home to care for it.

Malik wanted to become a rescuer. These courses regularly took place over a weekend, and there were about twenty to thirty people in each course. I loved animals, but I had no desire to spend a whole weekend learning about them. People, on the other hand...I could always spend time with people. So if Malik, who found people unnerving, needed a partner, I was 100 percent in.

"I'll go with you," I told him. "Let's do it!"

We humans need to develop an awareness of just how judgmental we can be. Our minds are quick to form negative thoughts and criticize. Sadly, the person we are usually the most negative about is...ourselves.

"What are three things that are great about you?" is a question I regularly ask young people when I meet them for counseling. I have come to expect the usual answers: "I'm great at gaming." "I'm good at soccer." "I'm pretty good at drawing." I then have to rephrase the question. "Those are three things that you are great *at*," I point out. "What about three things that are great *about you*?"

It's a hard question for anyone to answer. Most of us don't like to brag about ourselves. The first thing I hear from a young person's mouth is rarely "I'm kind" or "I have a great sense of humor" or "I'm creative." But they can always list their faults: "I'm a loser." "I'm not pretty enough." "I'm stupid."

Occasional self-doubt and self-criticism are a normal part of life, but constantly belittling yourself has a major impact on your self-confidence and mental health. It can cause depression, relationship difficulties, and problems with body image. We all have negative self-talk, but we should also be honest about our strengths. Being capable of recognizing your value is essential for your self-esteem.

One day, I was walking through the mall with my fourteen-year-old niece, and we passed a group of teenagers. I noticed her shoulders hunch slightly as she looked away from them. I was immediately reminded of being fourteen years old and full of self-consciousness. At this age, we think other young people are looking at us, sizing us up, and judging us. Being a teenager is horrendous.

During adolescence and puberty, we go through radical changes. The only other time our bodies, brains, and social and emotional development undergo such extreme shifts is in the first three years of life. Teenagers have to navigate the physical changes: the growing pains of bones lengthening and broadening, voices breaking or breasts appearing, and all that hair! There's a lot of checking yourself out in the mirror when you're a teenager, wondering whose body this is. But that is just the beginning. The brain of an adolescent is realigned; memories are shredded, logic goes out the window, and impulsivity goes through the roof. The brain is a hive of hormones and turbulent emotions. Adolescence is a mixed-up, messed-up, crazy time filled with insecurity and anxiety as teenagers examine and critique their own changing bodies and constantly compare themselves with others in a desperate bid to fit in. Teenage angst is real.

This type of social anxiety is a natural part of maturing, and most of us grow out of it. As we get older, we may care deeply about what other people think, but we become aware that not every person in our day-to-day interactions is thinking about us. Why would they be? Their heads are filled with their own busy lives.

No matter how confident or self-assured we are, we still have moments when we're afraid that people are judging us. Public speaking, for instance, is a fear almost everyone has.

I do a lot of public speaking. I present at conferences, run trainings, and do media interviews, and I still get nervous whenever I have to stand in front of a crowd. I need to pee several times in the half hour leading up to the event, and I get dry mouth every single time. My mind always goes straight to the negative: *What if I make a fool of myself? Will I sound smart enough? Do I have anything to say that anyone is even interested in? Will they think I'm completely incompetent?* (Yes, impostor syndrome runs deep.) These thoughts make my legs quiver and my tongue go pasty just as I need to get the words out.

But this is what social anxiety does. It plays tricks on the brain. It makes us scrutinize ourselves, and we invariably believe everyone is thinking the same negative thoughts about us that we are. We fear failure and convince ourselves that others think we are failing. We believe we can't live up to others' standards, that we're not good enough, or that we're boring. And when people have these thoughts, they stumble over words, and the notes in their hands begin to shake. Essentially, they get trapped in a self-fulfilling prophecy, becoming their own worst critics and losing all their confidence.

For many autistic people, the perception that everyone is thinking specifically about them can remain throughout their lives. While most neurotypical people develop an understanding that those they meet in their day-to-day brief interactions don't really think much about them, some autistic people don't grasp this. Social anxiety can be based in the thought that others are thinking about you *all* of the time.

Savanna came across as a confident and extroverted young woman, but she was always second-guessing herself. At eighteen years old, she dressed like a character in an anime series, with short skirts, big boots, and knee-length socks. She was easily delighted and prone to high-pitched squeals. She loved a party. It wasn't obvious that Savanna suffered from social anxiety, but while she loved spending time with people, it involved an onslaught of constant self-assessment.

"Am I talking too much? Will they find me over the top? Do they want me to shut up? They must think I am super-annoying and really don't like me!" Savanna rambled. She could be thinking all of this even in mid-conversation. "But when I get anxious and think these thoughts, I just talk even more!"

Everyone thought Savanna was so much fun—everyone except Savanna herself. We usually think of people who are outgoing as being confident in all situations, but sometimes they are "people pleasers" desperate for approval.

While Savanna talked up a storm to try to cover up her fear of judgment, Neela tried hard never to talk to anyone at all. Neela had been struggling with social anxiety for most of her life. At thirty, she still found walking in a public place a nightmare, so she always wore just one earbud.

"I have to listen to music when I am out," she explained. "It calms and distracts me. But wearing two earbuds freaks me out. I need to keep one ear open, because people could be talking about me."

Neela was self-conscious. She slouched and kept her eyes cast down. She wished she could blend into the background, unseen. She fretted about what others thought of her dress sense, her hairstyle, and the way she walked. She believed that everyone, including me, was staring at her and thinking negatively about her.

"Why are you judging me?" Neela said when she arrived at my office one day. "When I walked in, your eyes went up and down my body!"

"That wasn't judgment, Neela," I explained. "That was envy. I was thinking, *What a great outfit. I wish I had a sweater like that.*"

Neela's social anxiety was crippling. She struggled every time she had to speak to someone, and she never spoke up if something was wrong. "If I go out with my family and they order me a hamburger but the waiter brings nachos, I'll just eat the nachos," she said. "I'd never ask a waiter for anything, not even sugar for my coffee. I just won't ask. They'll think I'm a complainer or a fool for ordering the wrong thing."

The nervousness of being judged, feeling embarrassed, or being laughed at can be so severe that it brings on heart palpitations and stomach cramps. It seems easier to just stay home, doesn't it? This is how many autistic people move through the world. Social anxiety can stop people from going to school, work, and restaurants and even from eating in front of others. It can stop people from entering a room where anyone else is already seated or from ever raising a hand and asking for help.

Wouldn't our self-esteem benefit if we could stop our negative self-talk and see ourselves as strong and smart and worthy and so beautiful, Michelangelo should have sculpted us in stone? And wouldn't it be wonderful if instead of believing people were thinking the worst of us, we thought that everyone viewed us with unconditional positive regard?

The next time you get that thought in your head—the one that says you're not attractive enough, you're not strong enough, you're not good enough, that you are going to fail or make a complete fool of yourself—remember that nearly everyone around you is pretty much thinking the same thing about themselves.

* * *

Before Malik and I attended the wildlife-rescue course, I called and asked them a thousand questions so I could gauge the expectations for the weekend.

Would we have to do any presentations? Would we be in large or small groups? Could Malik and I work together? Would the assessment be written or verbal? Would we be examined? Appraised?

On Saturday, I picked Malik up at eight a.m. I was worried. Would he be okay? Would he get through the first hour? The first day? The whole weekend? Malik fretted the entire car trip: "I'm not smart enough to do this. I'm wearing the wrong shirt. I'm going to say something stupid. I'm not going to finish it. Everyone will hate me."

For the first few hours, Malik and I were joined at the hip. I couldn't take two steps without Malik taking them with me. He wouldn't introduce himself as we went around the room, so I did it for him. He kept his head down and wiped his palms on his jeans.

To my complete surprise, about three hours in, sitting in a room with twenty-six new people, Malik raised his hand.

"So, you're saying that if we see a dead kangaroo on the side of the road, we should stick our hand in its pouch to see if there's a live joey inside?" Malik asked.

"Yes," said the Steve Irwin–look-alike instructor.

"And if it's suckling, we cut the teat off because a furless joey is permanently attached to the teat?"

"Yes."

At the break, Malik spoke with several people about joey rescues. He talked about how baby kangaroos are born half an inch long and then blindly climb through their mothers' fur to the pouch, where they stay for at least six months. (How cool are marsupials?) He explained that kangaroos are perpetual mothers and produce two different kinds of milk at the same time, one for a tiny joey growing in the pouch and one for a joey who has left the pouch but still nurses. Malik was center stage, and the people around him were nodding and listening.

"Are you doing okay, Malik?" I asked after the break.

"Yes," he said. "All these people think about is animals! They're not thinking about me at all."

He participated all weekend. He spoke to people about red-bellied black snakes, fruit bats, and sugar gliders. He spoke about blue-tongued lizards, platypuses, and numbats. He volunteered when the teacher needed one and was the first to demonstrate rescue techniques — in front of the whole class.

Malik and I both graduated. I was pathetic as an animal rescuer and had to call the hotline to be taken off the volunteer contact list. I'm not responsible enough to have a baby wombat or sick magpie in my home. I had to admit to them that I am just more of a people person.

Malik, however, was a superstar. The rescue team learned to text him and not call. He would travel everywhere and show his wildlife-rescuer card to strangers who had reported a hurt animal. Malik had to talk to all sorts of people and record details of the injured animals. Then he would take the creatures home and care for them.

"So, you are saying echidnas are shy?" Malik had asked our khaki-wearing teacher. "And if you approach an echidna, it'll roll into a ball and show only its spines?"

"Yes."

"Or it'll dig itself into a hole and retreat to avoid contact?"

"Yes."

Malik turned to me and mouthed: *I am an echidna.*

I smiled and thought, *Maybe a little. But even if you think of yourself as spiky and strange, everyone else thinks that you're fascinating.*

# 27

# Pete's Door

Pete called me a bulldog, and I took this as the highest compliment.

Pete had a big tattoo on his upper arm of an eagle swooping down on its prey. He was broad-shouldered, sported a scruffy beard, and had a long ponytail. He was one of the most well-read people I had ever met, and he could discuss philosophy, sociology, and anthropology for hours on end. He knew something about everything but had very few people in his life with whom to share his knowledge.

By his mid-twenties, Pete had stopped engaging in all the services available to support people with disabilities — not that you'd immediately think he had one. At first glance, Pete didn't seem to need much support, but he had always struggled. He had attended mainstream schools but had had few friends and often battled with the school system. During his school years, he was deemed defiant, lazy, and confrontational. He therefore didn't last long in an environment set up for the neurotypical majority and was suspended multiple times before he dropped out completely.

Pete could drive a car, cook, clean, and budget. He lived at home with his mom and had no intention of ever moving out or even getting a job, for that matter.

"Why work your whole life and then die?" Pete had told the employment-center coordinator who was assessing Pete's employability. Though Pete had given work a go in the past, it had never been successful. Every time he had a job trial in a new workplace, he invariably knew more about the job than the boss, and he let them know it. He did not believe in hierarchical systems of management or in following the directions of a superior.

Pete believed that most people were either illogical or hypocritical. If someone crossed Pete's moral code or wasn't intelligent enough or did not follow through on exactly what they'd said they'd do, Pete erased them—forever. It didn't take long for Pete to drop people and services and supports. *No* was his response to any service referral.

When I first met Pete, he had been at home for months. He engaged with his immediate family and with others through online gaming, but not with anyone else. He stayed in his room all day and was totally disconnected from the outside world. When his mom booked him for appointments to see people like me, he didn't show. He refused to leave the house. He wouldn't even get out of bed.

So I went to him.

The first time I arrived, Pete stayed in his room and pretended to be asleep. I stayed in the house for the full hour of therapy and sat with his family. I knocked on his door twice that day, once to say I was there and once before I left. On leaving, I said that I would be there every week.

"I just thought I would let you know," I said. "I'll keep coming back."

And then I kept going, week after week. I knew that Pete

had an interest in Greek and Roman mythology, so I would knock on his bedroom door, sit on the floor next to it, and read aloud the tales of the gods. Sometimes he would yell at me and tell me to fuck off and go away. Sometimes he would say nothing at all; from the other side of that door, I'd have no idea whether he was listening or sleeping.

After nearly four months of weekly visits and floor-sitting, I arrived one day and nearly fell over myself when I saw him up, dressed, and in the living room.

"I never thought I'd meet someone more stubborn than me," he said. "You just won't give up, will you?"

What is trust?

> *I have never even thought about it. I just know it when it's there.*

> *You just know who you can trust and who you can't trust!*

> *It's about belief and faith, but it is also about hope.*

Trust is extremely important to all of us. It's said to be one of the central components of a relationship, yet if this is true, why is it so hard to put a finger on exactly what it is?

I am a very trusting person; I believe in the genuine good in people. I leave the house unlocked (don't tell the insurance agency) and I'm happy to have strangers stay, even when I'm not there. After my car was broken into, I started to leave it unlocked too. I placed twenty dollars in an envelope on the console and wrote on it, *There is nothing worth taking in this car, but if you need something, here is twenty bucks to help you out.* Strangely, no one ever took that envelope or broke into my car again.

My mother would say that I trust too easily. When I was nine years old, my brother and I were allowed to sit outside a department store in the small town where we lived while my mother was shopping. We sat on a bench and chatted to an old man. He was a nice old man who told us all about his life.

When my mom came out of the store, the first words out of my brother's mouth were "Mommmmmm, Jodi kissed an old man!" And it was true, I had. I'd felt sad for his saggy face, so when he said, "I have to go, give me a kiss," I puckered up my lips and laid one on that wrinkled, craggy old cheek of his.

That night I got a good talking-to. It wasn't an angry talk, just a this-is-so-serious-we-will-go-to-your-bedroom-and-discuss-this-away-from-your-siblings talk.

"Jodi, you don't have to do what people ask you to do, particularly strangers!" my mom said. "We don't kiss people that we don't know. We don't trust people until we get to know them."

I have needed to be reminded of this for most of my life. But I trust easily, and I believe that most of us *are* trustworthy, perhaps because this has seldom been disproven for me; I've been very fortunate in this regard.

But I have seen people I love lose trust. I've seen people I care for betrayed, and I have seen their confidence in humanity shattered. I have watched as friends have been lied to, have had their secrets revealed, and have had loyal "friends" turn their backs.

"When trust has been broken, it is almost impossible to recover," my friend told me. "You become wary, cautious, defensive. You tread very carefully." She raised both hands and showed me her ten fingers. "I can count on two hands the number of people I trust."

Silas could hold up only two fingers, representing his parents. Silas was a physics geek. I rarely understood anything he said in our appointments, and any discussion about physics was not really a discussion at all. Silas explained thermo-dynamics and electromagnetic waves and gravitational fields, and my brain ached trying to understand what he was saying. Silas had been referred to me for support in developing relationship skills, but this was another person's idea of what Silas wanted. Silas, in fact, wasn't at all interested in having friends.

"I like things that are consistent, things that are reliable" was how Silas explained it to me. "People are extraneous variables and, just as in science, these variables are confounding."

Silas was right. People don't fit into a neat control group. They all have shifting moods and personality types and can be temperamental and fickle at times, but most of us gravitate toward people who are steady and dependable.

When you trust someone, it is because that person has earned your trust. We don't just trust people willy-nilly (although some people may think I am a little lax on this front); we watch them and take note and check for consistent behavior. We wouldn't use a bathroom scale that goes up or down by five pounds one day to the next, and we all want a reliable car that gets us from point A to point B. It's the same with people. We feel safe and secure when we know a person will deliver on their promises. As Silas had complained to me, people say many things that they don't follow through on.

"People have been like this my whole life," he explained. "When I was a kid, someone would say, 'We'll go to the park today after school,' and I would think about that all day—and then we wouldn't go. Or they'd say, 'Yeah, you can come to my birthday party,' but then I wouldn't get an invitation. And adults are the worst. How many people have promised they would stay in touch and then they don't? It's all just empty words."

Think of how many times you say, "We have to catch up! I will text you," and then before you know it, you run into that person again and not once have you called or texted—and neither have they. We understand in these moments that life sometimes gets in the way, and we don't judge one another for not following through on our kind intentions. Silas didn't take this as lightly as most people do.

"I set up a screening process," Silas said. "If people break a promise, then I don't want them in my life. People should not make promises that they cannot keep."

One of the biggest promises you can make is that you'll keep a secret. It's one of the highest levels of trust you can place in someone. In my personal life, when someone says, "Please don't tell" or "Please keep this between us," it becomes classified information. But often they don't even need to say these words. Sometimes the weight and emotion of a story says it all: *This is mine and mine alone, and I am sharing it with you because I trust you.*

But not all secrets can be held. On the first meeting with any new client, I let them know this. I hold confidentiality in the highest regard in my work, but I am ethically and legally obligated to break the keeping-secrets rule if a person indicates they may harm themselves or others.

After I disclose this fact, I make it clear that for anything beyond that, my lips are sealed. Everything else they share with me is under lock and key.

Even if you promise someone that they can trust you with their secrets, and even if they believe you, it can still be very hard for people to talk about the things that hurt them the most. No matter how much you trust someone, revealing your innermost self can make you feel vulnerable.

Are there parts of yourself that you have never shared with anyone? Your deepest darkest secrets? A story from your past? Your regret, shame, or guilt? Your thoughts of hopelessness or your fears? Each of us has thoughts about the past, present, and future that we have placed in a sealed casket and buried as deep within us as we can. We push these thoughts deep down so that we don't have to feel them, reflect on them, or face them. If we have this much difficulty being open and honest with ourselves, how do we share our truth with others?

Different people have different relationships to trust. Trust is not one-size-fits-all.

Working with neurodivergent people, I have realized that it is profoundly important that relationships are built on their terms and within their time frames and that they're able to express themselves in their own way. Some people might say very little when we are face-to-face with them, but then send a long e-mail or text filled with deep musings, profound reflections, and disclosures that could not be said in person. The written word allows them to divulge their secrets in ways they cannot when we are together.

The words on the pages might read:

*Every time I am coming to see you, I lie in bed the night before and think, I'm going to tell her tomorrow. And then I come and the words get stuck in my throat...but the truth is...*

Or:

*I just don't feel it's something I can talk to you about just yet. It's a really heavy topic, I guess, and very, very exposing—I can feel myself getting embarrassed about it already.*

Or:

*I have a sort of confession and I've been feeling ashamed almost since we first met. I want to tell you, but I can't because if I do, then it will really be true.*

It takes a lot of courage to confront our demons out loud. Some of my clients like the "five-minutes-to-go" explosion. For forty-five to fifty minutes, there is everyday easy interaction or lots of "I don't know" answers to questions and then, *wham*— five minutes before the end of a session, the vulnerability of hurt, pain, and confusion is dropped like a glass on a tile floor. I always struggle in these moments. It takes longer than five minutes to sweep the shards and splinters into a neat pile, and how do we ever glue the glass back together? But I also understand the courage it has taken for these people to reveal themselves and the torment they must have experienced contemplating whether they could say their secret out loud. I always acknowledge their bravery. Showing vulnerability is the most fearless act of all.

Trust is essential in relationships, and being consistent, truthful, and patient and holding secrets are essential for building it. We all want people in our lives we can bank on, depend on, and rely on, those who say, "I have your back, I won't let you down, I'm here for you, you can rely on me." When we have these people, we hold on to them tight. Trust is built slowly, brick by brick by brick, and then this trust cements us together.

If one thing bound Pete and me, it was reliability. Pete left his bedroom, then his house, and eventually he started coming to see me in my office. Over the years, Pete continued to open his doors wider and wider.

"I just don't trust people," he told me. "I never have. You know how people say that you should give them the benefit of the doubt? Well, I always have doubt." He said that it was so much easier to avoid people than to be disappointed, so he shut them out. "It's much better that way—then no one ever lets you down."

"So why'd you give *me* the benefit of the doubt?" I asked. "Why did you finally come out of your bedroom?"

"Because you kept turning up." He laughed. "You just kept coming back, week after week. I realized that when you said, 'I'll keep coming back,' you meant it. You were so persistent."

"And how long did it take you to trust me? How long did it take you to feel like you could say anything and everything to me?"

"Three years. Trust is like Rome—it wasn't built in a day, Jodi."

I thought back to those first few months of sitting on the floorboards outside of Pete's closed door, reading tales from Roman mythology to him. It was a week-in, week-out statement of "I am here." Doors can get stuck; they can get off kilter and their hinges can sag. They need a solid, reassuring frame of support so that they can be opened. Kind of like people.

# 28

# Imogen's Eggs

Imogen loved eggs. Not fried or scrambled or poached, not the taste of them or the texture in her mouth. Imogen loved the feeling of eggs between her fingers. Raw eggs. It *is* an amazing feeling. Soft and soothing, slippery and sticky—and so sensual.

We try to find ways to connect with our kids. We play with them and read to them and hug them. We want our children to be happy. But when your child is different—when your child turns away from a hug, cannot remain still for a story, and has no interest in playing with toys—you search for the things that you both love and hope they will bring you together. So, just as eggs bond a cake, Imogen's mom used eggs to bond them together.

"I thought it would help us to develop a similar interest," her mom told me. "I thought if we could do something together, just one little thing, it would build our relationship."

So Imogen's mom taught her six-year-old daughter how to bake. They would stand together, side by side, at the kitchen island and create a concoction—a mud cake or a sponge cake or some biscuits. Together they would sift the flour and measure the sugar and pour the milk. And then came the eggs.

Imogen's mom would give her the eggs to crack, but to Imogen, the eggs were not part of the cake. They were not meant to be mixed with other ingredients—they were meant to be sloshed through her fingers. Imogen found something extraordinary in eggs. They felt like *bliss*.

And so the Egg War began.

At first, Imogen's obsession with eggs was annoying. Every chance she got, she would head to the fridge, open the door, and survey the shelves for her all-time-favorite thing. Once she found the eggs, she would crack them onto the kitchen floor and rub her hands in that soothing calm. Not just one egg; one was never enough. Imogen would take as many eggs as she could get her hands on. She would crack the shells, discard them to the side, then slide her hands and arms and body over the mess on the floor. For the family, this was a problem. (For one thing, they were going through *a lot* of eggs!)

Imogen's parents worked from home. They both became attuned to the sound of the fridge door opening. It created a Pavlovian response: they ran to the kitchen. Sometimes, Imogen's parents weren't fast enough to stop her from smashing the eggs onto the floor. "But I would stop in the middle of whatever I was doing and run," her mom told me.

Then one day, when her mom was in the middle of a laborious Excel spreadsheet, she heard the fridge open. *The eggs* was all she could think.

When she ran into the kitchen, there was Imogen. But she hadn't touched anything in the fridge; she was just holding the door open. Imogen went to her mother and took her by the hand.

That fridge door had become shorthand for *Hey, Mom, I need you. Hey, Mom, I need some help. Hey, Mom, look what I have done!*

*Hey, Mom, it is not about the eggs anymore. Hey, Mom, I have learned something new. Hey, Mom, I have learned that the fridge door will bring you to me. Hey, Mom, the fridge door connects us.*

Some people may not express their emotions in a clear way; some may not like to be hugged or look people in the eye. Some may speak a different language, echo words, ask the same question again and again, or use different gestures. Some people may reach out by sending more than three texts, or they may hide behind doors or pace or spin or flap their hands. Some will info-dump about locks and keys, lick others on the arm, smash an egg, or open a fridge door just to say *Be with me.*

*Humankind*—there is a reason why *kind* has been added to the word *human.* We need to rise to this challenge. All of us want to connect. We all want to belong. We try to do so in any way we can. Sometimes our attempts are clumsy or odd, and occasionally they're painful, but we try nonetheless. We need to open our minds and hearts to the multitude of ways we relate to one another. It is in recognition and celebration of our unique differences that connection and belonging are built.

So the next time you stand gazing out over a clover patch, remember that four-leaf clovers can always be found; you just have to believe in the brilliance of diversity. And open your eyes to see.

# Acknowledgments

Writing a book has been one of the most challenging and rewarding experiences of my life. I had thought that writing was a solitary pursuit, but this is far from the truth. Writing takes a team of people who support you, turn your words into a book, and turn you into a writer.

Tracy Behar, the most brilliant of editors. When I first met you, you held an imaginary book in your hands and made me believe it was possible. I cannot thank you enough for consistently hearing my voice, for your guidance, and your belief. I am forever grateful.

Georgia Frances King, my agent turned subeditor turned friend. You started this! When you called and I said, "I'm not a writer," you said, "Just give it a go." This book would not exist without you. I cannot begin to express my appreciation. Jane von Mehren, agent extraordinaire. Across the planet and through multiple time zones, you have been a constant source of wisdom. Thank you for championing me and for changing my life. There are some moments that live with you forever. For me, the moment when, out of my pure disbelief, you both cried because I cried is one of them.

To the team at Little, Brown Spark. Thank you all for your tireless work on the book. When I saw the beautiful cover, my first thought was *How can they know me so well?* It is perfect. And to Julianna's nephew: I hope your collection of clovers brings a lifetime filled with magic and adventure.

Thank you to everyone at Souvenir Press, particularly Cindy Chan, Publishing Director, for your support and enthusiasm.

Thank you to Nathaniel (Nate) Glanzman from Writing Diversely for your thoughtful reading and perceptive feedback through your lens of lived experience.

To the team at Northern Pictures, particularly Cian, Jenni, and Karina. Even though you didn't provide hair and makeup, I cannot thank you enough for the incredible experience of *Love on the Spectrum.*

Thank you, Mike, because you're the person I trusted most to read first. You've held all of my vulnerability but also didn't hold back on the slash-and-burn. I couldn't have managed the past few years without you . . . on every front! I'm really, really, really grateful.

Janice, thank you for early-morning walks and swims and for your fine art in constructive criticism. You're a lifesaver. Sharmi and Shaz, thank you for listening to me read out loud, which is always terrible, but you listened anyway. That in itself is a true reflection of our friendship. Jen, thanks for keeping me grounded and for opening my gills. I treasure all of you.

While writing I found I needed places where I could retreat and bury myself in words. For me there were two havens where I was able to do this.

I am so very grateful for Valla. The space, the people, the dogs, beach, stars, wood fires, and gardenias. And for Miles, thank you for every "This is random," for every "What's the word?," and for every single "You can, Jodes."

Thank you to everyone at Nusa Indah in Indonesia who shared Bintangs, sunsets, night swims, and stories with me, and to the staff who always put me in the same room. *Terima kasih untuk semua orang di Nusa Indah yang telah membantu saya selama saya menulis disana. Saya sangat bersyukur.*

I couldn't have written this book without the support of music. Our lives are enriched by artists. I particularly want to thank Bruce Springsteen because the story behind the creation of "Dancing in the Dark" was the push that kept me going. It became my earworm.

Thank you to every person I've had the pleasure of working with, my colleagues over the last thirty-odd years. I'm one of those very lucky people who wake up nearly every day wanting to go to work! Part of this is because of you.

And to all of *my* people...you know who you are, because you already know what you mean to me. Thank you for keeping me afloat when I struggled and for making me feel like I'm the player being hoisted onto your shoulders at the end of a game. My cup is always overflowing.

Sash and Indi...please know I'd take back this promise a trillion times over just to have your mum here. I'm so thankful you are both in my world.

And Sage, my beautiful daughter. Thank you for the illustrations and every part of you found in these pages. I love you more than everything I've done today. Every single day!

Mum and Dad, thank you for giving me a life filled with your constant encouragement and open expression of pride. I love that you are proud of the simple things—African violets, the backstep, and, although you will deny it, my fifty-year-old toaster.

To my family, all of you! I won the family lottery! Because of you, I know that joy, laughter, and unconditional love are free, real, and readily available. I know what the world feels like when there are always wide-open arms ready to gather you in. I love you.

Last but most, to the hundreds upon hundreds of autistic, neurodivergent, and disabled people and their families who I've been privileged to spend time with. You have taught me so much and given me a lifetime of stories. I'm a better person because of you. One book cannot express how grateful I am that, because of all of you, I'm living a full and fulfilled life.

# About the Author

Jodi Rodgers is a qualified counselor, sexologist, and special-education teacher with thirty years of experience in the education, disability, and sexuality fields. During her career, she has helped clients of all ages and their families, from early intervention to high schools and adult and community settings. She specializes in working alongside both disability and sexual-health organizations. Her private practice, Birds and Bees, helps neurodivergent people learn about the complex areas of sexuality and relationships and, even more fundamental, how to create love and connection. She has become well-known as the relationship counselor on the hit Netflix show *Love on the Spectrum*.